The Healing Journey of My Bodacious Ta Tas

Healed by Grace and on a Budget

Venus DeMarco
with
Lisa Smith

authorHOUSE®

AuthorHouse™
1663 Liberty Drive
Bloomington, IN 47403
www.authorhouse.com
Phone: 1-800-839-8640

In no event shall Venus DeMarco or its contributors have any liability for incidental or consequential damages relating to use of any of the information and ideas contained in this book.

All the information that I have shared in this book, is the truth as I know and have received it. My prayer is that you will take the time to find the truth as it applies to your own personal life.

© 2012 by Venus DeMarco

No part of this book may be reproduced, stored in a retrieval system, or transmitted by any means without the written permission of the author.

Published by AuthorHouse   11/06/2012

ISBN: 978-1-4772-7466-8 (sc)
ISBN: 978-1-4772-7464-4 (e)
ISBN: 978-1-4772-7465-1 (hc)

Library of Congress Control Number: 2012917966

Any people depicted in stock imagery provided by Thinkstock are models, and such images are being used for illustrative purposes only. Certain stock imagery © Thinkstock.

This book is printed on acid-free paper.

Because of the dynamic nature of the Internet, any web addresses or links contained in this book may have changed since publication and may no longer be valid. The views expressed in this work are solely those of the author and do not necessarily reflect the views of the publisher, and the publisher hereby disclaims any responsibility for them.

Annette
May this book bless you!
Jamie ?

Introduction

Let me ask you: is it the fear or the disease?

As serious as the subject of cancer is, *The Healing Journey of My Bodacious Ta Tas* will take you from laughter to tears with eyes wide open. Come along with me as I travel through the Disneyland of cancer treatment centers, to the Redneck Riviera, and over the borders of Mexico to discover the truth about healing. The road ahead would prove to be difficult at times. As a matter of fact, I ran into Goliath along the way and had to gather up enough courage to stand face to face with him.

But it was in the midst of my search for answers, with fear breathing down my neck, that blind faith taught me to say it was really over from the moment that I was diagnosed. I just didn't realize it. Healing is a gift from God, and I have found that practicing good nutrition is a wonderful path that allows me to live a long, healthy, and productive life. My story will inspire other women not to become their disease, and if ever diagnosed with cancer, the chance to have peace of mind much sooner than I did. Learning the truth does set you free!

I am not a celebrity or a wealthy individual. I am a single, self-employed woman in my 50s in an economical situation that many people today share. Since the diagnosis, I have been speaking to various groups throughout the United States on the topic question, "Is it the fear, or the disease?" I also encourage those who have decided to take the natural route versus the conventional route. My website, www.venusdemarco.org, contains information for those who are seeking knowledge to live a healthier life, including recipes, blogs, and a nutritional supplement store.

Soon after I was diagnosed, I began talking about the book that I was going to write which would take the fear out of women's hearts. This book is for anyone who has breasts, or for those who simply enjoy an inspirational story.

My Prayer is this book will lead to more conversations about the potential for cancer and disease prevention through lifestyle changes. But more than anything that it takes the FEAR out of your hearts when it comes to CANCER!

Sincerely,
Signature
Venus DeMarco

Dedications

Living this journey and writing this book has forever changed my life, and I would love to thank the following people for all they did in their own special way.

Gayle, for being there from the beginning, always helping me spiritually, emotionally, and even financially. I will never be able to thank you enough. To Teresa Tapp for believing in me from the start even when you didn't really know me. Thank you so much for giving me my first speaking gig to tell my story. You awoke the beast. Most of all, for your belief in this book. Lisa, without you and your ability to sit me down, listen, and record my whole story, I don't know if it would have ever gotten done. Thank you for helping me get this on paper. I will forever be grateful. Charlotte, for kicking me in the butt to get this thing started. To my sister, who I love more than anyone in the world. I know this wasn't easy for you especially because at first you didn't understand what I was doing. To Brenda, Janelle, and all the Ta Ta Sisterhood—you know who you are—just know I hold all of you close to my heart. Jan, Pilar, and Cindy, for calling me every day for at least two years, to see how I was doing, encouraging me, and praying for me. God Bless you. Pilar, for the many Whole Foods' gift cards. Victor, for your friendship and love. Even when you were in Afghanistan, you were always there. To my wonderful clients and friends, who took this bumpy road with me and didn't leave. Thank you! To my Aunt Joe and Aunt Nancy, you two wonderful people. Pam, thank you for just being you. Cathy De Marco, I feel like you are my other sister. Shelly, for spending your birthday with me. What a night! And then bringing Hot Al and Sophia to Austin for Thanksgiving. We are friends for life, that's what you always say.

Last but not least, thank you to my lovable, quirky Iggy.

Contents

Introduction	v
Dedications	vii
Good Friday	1
Blind Faith	23
The Disneyland of Cancer Treatment Centers	36
Redneck Riviera	46
Mexico or Bust	57
Home Sweet Home	65
A Year of Discovery	70
Everybody wants to be a Healer	77
Saint Janelle and the TaTa Sisterhood 2010	84
Defeating Your Goliaths	90
Is It the Fear or the Disease?	105
Remarkable Paths	113
Laughter	127
If I Had to Do It Over Again	131

Good Friday

As I wake up to another gorgeous day in Austin, Texas, I glance over to see my handsome dog Iggy asleep in his bed. It's at that very moment before my feet hit the floor, that I take time to tell God how grateful I am. For the last two years, I have consistently started my day off by thanking God for healing me and showing me that I am a victor, not a victim. I cannot begin to tell you the depth of strength, courage, wisdom and grace that He has filled my heart with.

April 10, 2009 *I hear the words that bring instant fear to so many people: "Venus you have breast cancer." Shockingly enough, it is no surprise to me. You see this very large mass that is approximately 9 centimeters has been there for almost six months. When it was obvious that the mass was abnormal, I asked my sister, who is a personal trainer, if I had pulled a muscle in my breast. She said, "Venus, you know that muscle isn't on top of the breast."*

The year and a half prior to that day, I had started doing a wellness program called T-Tapp. T-Tapp is a method of movement that is a compound muscle workout. This means it uses the full length of the muscle plus supporting muscles at the same time—full fiber muscle activation. It's neurokinetic, meaning it connects your mind to your body. Like the old saying, "Use it or lose it," this exercise keeps the mind youthful. Most important to me though, it's a Lymphatic workout. It stimulates lymphatic flow, which optimizes the lymph system. This means it moves waste out at a cellular level. The lymphatic system takes the trash out. I had enjoyed it so much that I was studying to be a trainer.

I was in Houston participating in a T-Tapp workshop in which we worked out for four hours straight. I felt great even though I was experiencing a terrible time with hot flashes.

That night I remember waking up at 4 a.m. from a rash on my arms. The bumps were white with red dots and covered both arms from the shoulder to the middle of my biceps. Strangely the rash didn't itch. I just thought that the workout I had been doing triggered the rash. However, I had been experiencing a lot of pain in my right breast when I lay on my side or flat on my stomach, in addition to the rash. So, I knew something wasn't right.

I had always heard that breast cancer wasn't painful and that the lumps were round like marbles or shaped like a hard pea. The mass on my breast was completely opposite of those descriptions. It was long and tubular in appearance and extremely painful at times. That being said, six months is a long period of time to ignore symptoms like mine. It wasn't that I was in denial; I just wasn't quite ready to do anything about it.

The time finally came when I was ready to address the symptoms that were affecting my bodacious Ta Tas. I scheduled an appointment with a nurse practitioner to get a referral for a mammogram. They quickly determined that something was wrong and rushed me to the ultrasound room. It was right out of one those old prison movies—the good prisoners are released for some recreation, while the ones who are in trouble are returned to their cells. It was crystal clear which patients were potential prisoners of breast cancer. That's for sure. There we waited in the ultrasound cell with the blank look of fear on our faces.

After a long and painful ultra sound, the radiologist came into the room and was frantically animated as she told me they had found a very large mass on my breast. Like I hadn't noticed. The only good thing she said to me during my appointment was, "Venus, at least there's always hope."

Once she left the room, I mentioned to the ultrasound technician that the radiologist really should consider a career change; she would be a great kindergarten teacher due to her excessive drama skills. She could keep kids entertained for long periods of time.

As I left the doctor's office that afternoon, I remembered walking out to my car feeling scared and afraid. I was all a lone. I sat there crying, not knowing what to do next. I did the only thing I knew to do; I headed back to my office to work. But, I couldn't work in this state of mind. Shock was dropping by to pay me a visit, a very handy mechanism of the body that allows you to handle things before you lose it. Once I made it to the office, I knew I had to cancel my clients for the remainder of the day. I was in need of some shoulders to cry on. I sat down at my desk to call my sister and a few close friends to share the news.

Before heading home, I received a call from the nurse practitioner, who had written the referral for the mammogram. She informed me that the radiologist urged me not to waste any time in scheduling an appointment with a cancer specialist. I did not allow her scare tactics to overwhelm me. Instead I informed her that I would get back to them next week. I knew I needed some time to think things through thoroughly because my mind was a train wreck of thoughts and emotions.

It really just blows me away how the medical society immediately upon diagnosis tries to instill fear in you. In fact, everyone around me was reacting out of fear. Not one person thought to ask me what I wanted to do. I cannot express to you enough: Do not get caught up in the fear! Is it fear or the disease? Keep this thought in your heart as you continue to read the chapters ahead.

The diagnosis was delivered to me on Good Friday, which is a very significant day to all Christians. It was on this particular day that our Lord and Savior, Jesus Christ, died to bring us hope and a new life. Isaiah 53: 5 – *"But He was wounded for our transgressions, He was bruised for our guilt and iniquities; the chastisement [needful to obtain] peace and well-being for us was upon Him, and with the stripes [that wounded] Him we are healed and made whole."*

I would eventually see this day as a day for me to get a new life, a new beginning in my health, mind, and soul. But for me to get there, it would be my faith that would be a very valuable commodity. What I needed right then more than anything was support and encouragement. I decide to call my dear friend Pam and ask her to stop by later on, bearing gifts of good food and red wine. Yes, I still wanted to eat! Nothing kills my appetite, not even being diagnosed with cancer. Don't tell me that food isn't comforting. You can't take the Italian out of the girl!

Upon arriving home that afternoon, I called my friend Jan, who lives in California and is a really strong Christian believer. I knew I needed to surround myself with people who would love me and offer positive reinforcement to me. She advised me to get in touch with a man named Eli and his wife Judy, so that they could pray and be in agreement for my healing.

Eli is an anointed man of God, who has an incredible gift of healing. The Bible says in Matthew 18:19 (NIV) - *"Again, truly I tell you that if two of you on earth agree about anything they ask for, it will be done for them by my Father in heaven."* I wasted no time in contacting them and asking them for prayer concerning my health. I found it so amazing that I could pick up the phone and call someone I didn't even know and have them stand in agreement with me for my healing. I cannot begin to tell you how special and important this was to me. Even though I was still in the state of shock, I knew right at that very moment my healing began.

As the news continued to spread, most of my friends just couldn't believe this was actually happening to me. I was the one, who always ate organic, took my supplements religiously and exercised consistently. But what we think is healthy just may not necessarily be.

Before I knew it, there was a knock at the door and it was Pam with food, wine, some liquid minerals, and a new boyfriend. My friend Pam, what an awesome woman she is. She's a little blonde New Zealander and is as passionate about health as I am. If you need Pam, she is always there. Sometimes she arrives so quickly that you would think she had transported herself (beam me up Pam). This time though, I remember thinking, "Wow! What a great time to meet a new boyfriend." The real kicker was that his wife had died from breast cancer, or as I prefer to say, from the treatment of cancer.

I had this strange man staring at me in fear and probably reliving some terrible memories in his mind. There I was in shock and as white as a ghost, trying to make him feel comfortable and at ease. But wait, wasn't I the one who was just diagnosed with breast cancer? We women are so nurturing, even in the midst of our very own crisis. It's just what we do. Once we all gathered ourselves, we ate, drank and discussed some natural ways of healing and how passionate we were about them.

After bidding Pam and her new boyfriend goodbye, I went over to see my good friend, Gayle, and we sat on her balcony with our dogs relaxing and enjoying the rest of the evening. As we sat there, we began to discuss my health. Gayle very calmly said the best thing a friend could have ever said, with absolutely no fear in her eyes. "Venus, you are going to be alright." She has been my friend, my cheerleader, and a shoulder to cry on throughout this entire journey. What would I have done without my dear friends?

Finally the moment came that evening, when I was alone with nothing but my thoughts and the diagnosis that lingered so loudly in my head. I remember going to bed that night, cuddling up with my dog and crying. Iggy never sleeps on the bed with me, but he knew that night I really needed him by my side. It would indeed prove to be a sleepless night.

I gave up the battle of trying to get some rest and got up around 4 a.m. I immediately found myself on the computer searching for any possible natural cures for breast cancer. I had no idea how this was going to change my life viewpoint on how I defined healthy. I found more information on the benefits of eating raw living foods than any other options. There have been times in my past that I have thoroughly enjoyed eating at raw food restaurants. But, I actually never thought about becoming a raw food enthusiast. Was I going to be a hippie again, wear dreadlocks and give the peace sign all day? Did I have to give up makeup, not shave my pits or legs too?

I have been a vegetarian a couple of times in my life, however, I didn't really benefit from it as much as I could have because I consumed too many refined carbs and soy products, which isn't actually healthy.

The information that I found on the raw vegan diet was very appealing to me. The food can be as gourmet as you want it and very flavorful as well. A raw vegan diet consists of no animal products, dairy, refined sugars, or gluten and the food is never heated above 115 degrees Fahrenheit. This method of preparation allows our foods to keep all the enzymes, micronutrients, and antioxidants alive instead of depleting our food of the nutrients we really need.

The Bible is very specific in telling us the importance of taking good care of our bodies. In 1 Corinthians 6:19-20 – *"Do you know not that your body is a TEMPLE of the Holy Spirit, who is in you, whom you have received from God? You are not your own; you were bought with a price. Therefore HONOR God with your body."* I really did—and still do—want to bring honor to God by taking care of my body better than I had in the past.

I made the commitment to give up sugar and to follow the raw vegan diet for the first six months after the diagnosis. After that period of time, I followed the raw vegan way of eating 80 percent of the time, allowing myself the other 20 percent to add cooked foods that I felt my body needed. I also allowed myself to enjoy the occasional treat. I only ate raw desserts though because refined sugars could not be a part of my diet.

I learned that cancer cells do not breathe oxygen. They are anaerobic cells, and they love sugar. In fact, a cancer cell has six to thirteen times more insulin receptors than a healthy cell has, because it is not breathing oxygen anymore; it is fermenting sugar. It lights up the cancer cells, gives it energy and can multiply it.

One of the first things I had to do was to get my kitchen in order so that I could prepare raw living foods properly. I needed to add some additional appliances to the food processor I already owned. I invested a few bucks in a VitaMix blender, which is the lawnmower of blenders. It can break down anything and is great for preparing green smoothies. The other two items I added were a good juicer and a dehydrator that have done wonders for my health. I feel and look so much better since I changed my way of preparing and eating food. I can honestly say that I have found the food to be absolutely delicious, filling, and most of all very satisfying.

I was successfully on my way to detoxing and healing my body as God gave me wisdom and insight. Proverbs 2:10 (Amp) – *"For skillful and godly Wisdom shall enter into your heart and knowledge shall be pleasant to you."* I knew that this was a journey not an overnight adventure. I was asking God to reveal wisdom and knowledge that would point me in the right direction every single step of the way.

I set aside time to educate myself about supplementation to alkalize my body, to reduce inflammation, and kill cancer stem cells. I also added daily shots of wheatgrass to my diet—and removed the weekly shots of tequila, just kidding, but maybe not. Let me repeat myself, this did not happen overnight; it is a journey. You cannot do something for two to three days or even a week and expect to get the results you are looking for and need. Stick with it, and I promise you will see results.

But back to the weekend I was diagnosed… I spent Saturday in a complete daze. On Easter Sunday I was invited over to my friends', Janelle and Kyle's, for our annual adult Easter Party. Now keep in mind that stress affects everyone very differently. After having a few cocktails—no, I hadn't arrived at the no alcohol state yet—I was feeling no pain, yet was trying to cover up excessive emotional pain I was carrying on the inside.

I found myself in the front yard hanging out when I decided, or should I say, I was determined to see the neighbor's—Tim and Damen—two basset hounds. I asked Tim, "Can I see your dogs?" He said no because Damen had hurt his back and was resting. I don't have a clue as to what possessed me to do what I did at that moment, but right there in the front yard, I took my shirt off. "Does this change your mind," I asked. He then reminded me that he was gay.

Stress does crazy things to people! Every Easter, my friends love to bring this up. They joke and say, "Yeah Venus, it's all about the Ta Tas." I don't think I will ever live this one down.

My old habits were beginning to re-surface again. I was resorting to what I knew; drinking to de-stress and partying to cover up the pain. However, I knew that I had to make some serious changes in the way I was living my life. I have always loved the Lord, but there have been times in my life that I didn't include Him with me on my journey. I was doing what I knew to do allowing my humanness to prevail. I knew it was time to get myself together and to get serious about this diagnosis.

I am including some of me, being real, in this book no matter how offensive or over the top it may seem. I realize that this book may not meet the so-called "proper" guidelines for some Christians. However, I have decided that I am going to tell the raw truth about my experience no matter what. I had to deal with a lot of stuff before I was ready to get down to business.

April 19, 2009 *I am headed to Shoreline Church where I have been attending for about six months. As service starts and the worship music begins, this overwhelming feeling of desperation begins to set in. I know I need something miraculous from God. The time comes in the service where they invite people who have requests forward to pray with the prayer partners. I have never done this before and it is completely out of my comfort zone. But I realize, especially in the face of something like cancer, the importance of stepping outside of your comfort zone.*

I ask Gayle who is sitting next to me to go down and pray with me. As we approach the prayer partner, my friend shares that the radiation machine called a Mammogram has found a lump in my breast. All I can do is stand and cry.

Returning to our seats, I feel an incredible amount of peace hovering over me and a calmness that is so welcoming.

On that day, I didn't realize it at the time, but I had met someone who would end up being very important to me on the journey that lay ahead. And I would have never met her if I had just stayed in my seat. Again I'll say step out of your zone!

April 20, 2009 *I am off to my first appointment with a cancer specialist, and I just know that today is the day I am going to receive a clean bill of health. The waiting room is filled with somber faces, but not me. I am with my friend Andrea Wells, and we are, odd as it may seem, laughing and making jokes. If you haven't heard, the body can't heal without joy. I know you've heard before that laughter is the best medicine. It's true.*

Proverbs 17:22 (Amp) – "A happy heart is a good medicine and a cheerful mind works healing, but a broken spirit dries up the bones." I know that I have to laugh and find joy in order for my body to heal.

The next thing I remember about that day is when the nurse called my name and led me to the examination room. I'd like to point out that I carefully selected a female doctor thinking that she would be much more compassionate than a male physician. Turns out, sex plays no part in the role of "cancer doctor."

Mistake number one, I allowed "Dr. Do-little for me" to do a needle biopsy, which would be a decision that I would come to regret down the road. If I had only known what I know now, I would have never permitted this procedure to happen.

You see a tumor is a calcified mass that encapsulates cancer cells to protect the body. Inside of a tumor can be cancer cells, but the tumor itself is not cancerous. By sticking a needle into a tumor it can cause the cancerous cells to spread throughout the body into the blood stream and lymph system therefore upping the chances of metastasizing the cancer. This is commonly referred to as tumor spillage.

Before leaving, the doctor said she would call me with the pathology results as soon as they came in. She told me she was certain that the mass was cancerous, recommending a mastectomy and chemotherapy. I looked at her and firmly told her, "NO, you will not!" She completely ignored my response telling me to make an appointment with her nurse for a PET Scan, which cost $2,000. It also has such an extreme amount of radiation that they advise you not to be around small children or pregnant women after this procedure. Could I even go home and be around my dog?

The cancer specialist called me the next day to confirm that the test results were positive. Oh and let me add that the doctor left this detailed information on my voice mail. Isn't that illegal? She reminded me again to make an appointment for the PET Scan. Why does the medical society think you don't have any say over your own body, and why did she keep pushing this in my face? Money? Power? Control? These were honestly the only answers I could come up with.

The next day I found myself Googling slang words for breast. To my surprise I ended up writing down over 138 variations. For example: airbags, bazookas, boobs, chesticles, cupcakes, dairy pillows, devils' dumplings, fun bags, hooters, hood ornaments, jugs, knockers, rib bumpers, tits, and this is just to name a few of my favorites. We all love them; beautiful mounds of flesh, fat and glands, so, why would I want to lose them? They are a part of me, and yes, part of being a woman, whether they are AA or EE. They are part of my God given body and I'm going to keep my bodacious Ta Tas.

I called and informed the not-so-compassionate doctor that she was fired. I refuse to be a dollar sign! Breast cancer is BIG money. Let me say it again, breast cancer is BIG money! Each patient makes the medical field between $800,000 and $1million dollars each year. In reality, where is the incentive to find a cure for cancer? If the real cure makes very little money and doesn't make or keep you sick, why would the medical field even want to find a cure?

April 23, 2009 I am an Esthetician with my own private skincare business. It is a typical workday for me, except for my roller coaster-like emotions. One minute I am slowly climbing to the top and the next I am plummeting to the bottom at break neck speed! It has been some ride these past few weeks.

That particular day, as I began preparing for my appointments, I remember being full of overwhelming anger and rage that this was happening to me. I was so mad that I took my arms and with one big swipe threw everything off my desk. Of course immediately following, I proceeded to climb under my desk, curl up in a ball, and weep.

A few minutes later my client arrived for her appointment to find me still underneath my desk. Thank God she was someone who knew me. She kept saying, "Venus, you don't have to work on me today." I insisted that I had to.

I couldn't afford not to work. My business was relatively new and who else would support me, but me? What complete insanity, having to work? But If I had retreated to a corner of my home and let everything go, I could have lost all my clients and my business. This painted a vivid picture for me, and I could honestly see how some people wind up homeless in situations like these. I can see it now, Iggy and I on the corner with a sign saying, "Lost everything to Fear not the Disease." At least Iggy is cute; he would have enticed the people passing by to contribute to our cause.

The first thirty days after being diagnosed are the most crucial to receive the support of family and friends. Instead of my family coming right away, they decide that they will wait until I had surgery, assuming that I was going the conventional route. Family and friends, wake up! The emotional toll this has on a person is overwhelming, and no one, absolutely no one should have to face it alone. My mother, whom I love dearly, didn't even come to see me in the beginning when I needed her the most.

My mind was intoxicated and spinning with an array of emotions such as shock, fear, sadness, and denial. You are not at a place to make any major decisions regarding your health for the first thirty days after being diagnosed. I highly recommend that you find a nice relaxing place and go away to allow yourself to destress and detox before you make any final decisions. Surround yourself with people who love and support you. It is important that you separate yourself from fear and the fear of your loved ones as well. Fear is frenzy, everybody feeds off of it, and when that happens, you can't think straight.

I continued to find the results of the diagnosis and the behavior of the medical field a hard pill for me to swallow. Many times I was on my knees crying hysterically. And yes, there were a lot of tears along the way. When you find someone trying to take something away from you, you wind up blaming. I blamed my breasts. One time I was in the shower and I recall this feeling of hate toward them, not wanting to touch or wash them. I blamed them for my pain. But logically, they had done nothing to cause this disease.

At this point of my journey, I had not yet learned to rest and trust in God as I should. When feelings of isolation and fear would crowd my mind inside the four walls of my home, I would wind up on the floor crying and asking God for wisdom. But that night, something so mind-boggling occurred. As I was on my face and knees in a fetal position with Iggy by my side, I cried out to God telling him, "If this is what I have to walk through, then help me to make the very best of it."

A sudden calm came over me that hushed the fear and noise inside of my heart. At that moment, I heard God speak to me as if He were standing right beside me, "Child, you are going to write a book and take the fear out of women's hearts." I certainly hope out of some men's hearts too. I said, "Really God? Did I hear you correctly?" That was the furthest thing from my mind at that moment. But yet instantly, I knew what the title of the book would be. Will anyone really believe what just happened to me?

I agreed to the challenge and asked God to put the right people in my path and provide me with the information I would need for the journey ahead. I was finally beginning to understand what others meant when they said God spoke to them. This was a pivotal turning point in which I decided right then and there to become a human guinea pig in order to find out what good and bad treatments were available for breast cancer. It would be a mission to discover the truth.

I *contacted the* modern cancer treatment facility in Texas that is supposed to be the "best of the best" and made an appointment for a second opinion. I was going to see what the fuss was all about. I didn't want anyone to say that I was lying about the diagnosis I was given at my first appointment. Notice that I do not say *my* diagnosis or *my* breast cancer. I do not claim the diagnosis as *mine*, and I refuse to own it.

I knew I had a lot of research to do between then and my appointment. I didn't want to walk in blind, but rather educate myself as much as possible. See, sometimes what you see is not the truth. And, I already knew I was healed.

May 13, 2009 *I am fully aware when I get to the cancer treatment center it will be a real test of my faith. It's Sunday morning and time for church. As service begins, I feel desperate even though I know the route that I am going to take. As they call the prayer partners forward, something comes over me. I am barreling down the aisle pushing people out of my way. I am determined to get to the same prayer partner who had prayed for me last week.*

Success.

She speaks to me and calls me by name. I am amazed that she remembers who I am. I tell her that the test results have been confirmed and the diagnosis is breast cancer. She looks at me and asks, "Venus, what are you afraid of?"

I am afraid of the doctors.

As we prayed that day, the peace that only comes from God was very present and real to me. Philippians 4:7 (NIV) – *"And the peace of God, which transcends all understanding, will guard your hearts and your minds in Christ Jesus."* Isaiah 26:3 - *"Thou wilt keep him in perfect peace whose mind is stayed on thee."*

For me it was an in and out thing, fear, no fear, fear, no fear. But when I wasn't fighting fear, I was almost elated. Whenever I prayed or was prayed upon, I always felt an incredible measure of peace and a sense of bravery that helped me in moving forward. If you haven't heard before, prayer really does work.

After the service I connected with Lisa, the prayer partner, to tell her what I had decided to do—I was going for a second opinion. She told me that when she prays for people, she doesn't usually blurt out such an insensitive question... "Venus, what are you so afraid of?" I told her that no one had asked me what I was afraid of. Most people would assume that I was afraid of the disease, but in actuality, I was afraid of the doctors. God knew exactly what I needed that day, and I am so thankful that He connected Lisa and my paths. There was an instant bond between us; it was as though we had known each other a long time. I didn't want to take advantage of her, but I knew I needed her prayers and support.

She provided me with some resources that she felt might be helpful. One of the books she gave me was *Healed of Cancer* by Dodie Osteen. The book was a beautiful story about how God healed Dodie after being sent home with liver cancer and only two weeks to live. She chose not to accept the diagnosis and prayed for two solid years for a clean bill of health. It has been over thirty years and Dodie is still declaring the faithfulness of God!

I repeat this scripture every day, Deuteronomy 28:61 – *"Cancer is a curse of the law..."* And according to Galatians 3:13 – *"Christ redeemed us from the curse of the law; therefore I am redeemed from cancer."* The word redeemed means to pay off, to fulfill, to set free of ransom. In other words, Jesus paid the debt on the cross for all diseases saving us from the curse of the law. I continue to repeat this every single day, all day long, knowing that this affliction will never come upon me again.

My faith was blind, though my eyes could not yet see the results of my healing. I choose to put all my trust in God's faithfulness and allow Him to be my great Physician. II Corinthians 5:7 – *"We walk by faith, not by sight."* I knew that by doing this, I was going to be OK. That doesn't mean I didn't experience some very dark moments, I just didn't stay there. I would pull myself back up to stand firm in faith and be reminded of the hope that I have in Christ. I fully believed that my new life was on the horizon. Each step of this journey would indeed prove be a true test of my faith.

May 18, 2009 *Kris Carr is my new inspiration. I ran across a DVD she composed called* Crazy Sexy Cancer. *She had been diagnosed with a rare, incurable cancer and was told by her doctors that there was nothing they could do. She went home, educated herself, and set out on a journey to discover everything she could about the natural approach to health and healing.*

How impressive! I want to do what the healthy girl is doing. She has not lost her hair or poisoned her body. And she's made it through challenges like detoxing her body and her spirit.

This is my confirmation. I've decided to take God's natural path for my healing.

I continued to read and educate myself with anything I could get my hands on. In the meantime, I corresponded with a lady named Lauren, who worked at T-Tapp. She said, "Venus I have met this amazing doctor who offers oxygen treatments to cancer patients and he looks just like Santa Claus."

I immediately responded to the lead and contacted Dr. Cotter. He listened very attentively as I shared my story with him and plans to get a second opinion. He was a very caring man, and he expressed his concerns to me about going to the cancer treatment center. I told him not to worry that he was my next stop after going to this facility in Texas, and reassured him that I was one strong, feisty Italian woman and I would be ok.

In retrospect, I completely understand the concerns he had. He was afraid that when the doctors pressured me, I might give in and go the conventional route. But I had to know what women went through when they were diagnosed. Why do women cut their breast off within forty-eight hours of being diagnosed? It didn't make sense to me.

I had no idea that this would be one of the hardest battles I would face because of all the things that would come against me. I think Satan and his little demons were jumping for joy when they heard I was going for a second opinion. We're going to get her, my little pretty and scare the pants off of her. But thank God for the strength, courage, and peace with which He would constantly sustain me.

Romans 16:20 – *"The God who brings peace will soon defeat Satan and give you power over him."*

Blind Faith

We focus not on what is seen, but on what is unseen.

May 2009 Why is it that some people get healed and others don't? Is their faith weak? Or does fear cause them to run into the arms of a doctor that is pressuring them with scare tactics? My faith is blind. I cannot see my healing, yet I believe that I am healed. I still see and feel the landmark where cancer has tried to set up camp on my breast. Yet I know, yet I trust, and yet I believe what I know to be true and that is God's faithfulness and the work that was completed at the cross. II Corinthians 5:7 – "We live by faith not by sight."

Blind faith to me is a personal belief that does not rest on any logical or material proof. Though I cannot see the results yet, I believe I am healed. That's my story, and I am sticking to it.

I know that cancer is not from God. If Jesus died on the cross not only for our sins but for our sickness too, then how are we sick? That doesn't make any sense to me. In Psalm 103:2 &

3 (Amp) – *"Bless the Lord, O my soul, and forget not [one of] all His benefits. Who heals [each one of] all your diseases."* Have we forgotten the meaning of the cross? I want to remind you as you are reading this that every disease known to mankind was nailed to the cross and the prescription to your sickness is Jesus.

Even though I know many Christian women who really love the Lord dearly, I ask this question: Where is their faith? It appears to me they put their faith into doctors instead of God. They say God will carry me through, but what does that really mean? That God is going to get them through the cruelty of cutting off body parts, the poisoning of chemo, and the burning of radiation? This is where I get confused and I see this as a conflicting belief. Why would you let someone harm you to get you better, yet believe that God will heal you from the damage the doctors have done. Wouldn't it be easier to trust God from the beginning and not move ahead without Him? Perhaps if some women would have just waited thirty more days, they might have received their healing.

I have spoken to many women both believers and non-believers since being diagnosed. I have found that the majority of Christian women are not open to hearing what I have to say about conventional treatment vs. God's natural way of healing. It's the non-believers that are more open to the limitless possibilities of our God.

Just because you see something doesn't mean it's the truth. I could have looked at my deformed breast from the tumor and given up a long time ago. Instead, I have been consistently walking in blind faith for over two years now. I have known and trusted God from the beginning that I was going to be ok. Yes, it would have been nice to see instant results, but it didn't happen that way for me. Sometimes faith is a testing of time. Hebrews 11:1 (NIV) – *"Now faith is confidence in what we hope for and assurance about what we do not see."*

It took over two years for Dodie Osteen to get her medical clean bill of health even though she had already received her healing two years prior. She was sent home to die and given a couple of weeks to live. Thank God it has now been over thirty years since that diagnosis, and she is still living life to its fullest. I have seen some people receive their miracle on the spot, while watching others walk it out like me.

I believe that the tumor in my breast didn't dissolve to my eyesight immediately because there was so much for me to learn. If you get results right away, you may not appreciate the other benefits that come to you during your journey of walking it out. I would have never learned the things I did, nor met all the people I needed to meet or experience the beauty of forgiveness and healing in the way that I did. Now, God can use all the information He has poured into me to help others along the way. There was a bigger picture that I couldn't see when I was diagnosed.

We live in a society that is driven by instant gratification. We get sick and we immediately run off to the doctor. Who knows how long the sickness has been growing, maybe for years. But we want instant results especially when it comes to cancer. We automatically hear the word cancer and we think it's a death sentence, and the drama begins in our mind.

When you are first diagnosed, you can't run to the doctor every thirty days or even ninety days to check for change. No one sticks to protocol long enough. Over testing in a short period of time is one of the biggest mistakes I see people make. When you do this it opens the door to fear.

I fully understand and comprehend the vastness that fear can play when you are first diagnosed. But the strange thing is that I can't remember it anymore. Logically I can and I know that I was very scared in the beginning. But God gave me a beautiful gift of peace that completely showered my heart and mind taking away every ounce of fear that lay within me.

Looking back, it's really hard to believe that I can't actually remember the feelings of fear anymore. There were many times of great darkness in the beginning where fear tried to makes its home in my mind, but I kept fighting it with the word of God. As my Pastor says, "Don't exchange what you do know for what you don't know." I knew that God said I was healed, and I also knew the importance that nutrition would play to help me get better. So I refused to exchange these two valuable things for something I didn't know.

It took me a good solid year to arrive where I am today, and it's so amazing to know that I do not have to ever experience that feeling of fear again. If you asked me to give you a comparison I would say it reminded me of stories of childbirth—painful during labor, but you will forget about the depth of pain when you are holding that beautiful child in your arms. That's how I feel about the fear. Press through the fear; choose to trust God, and I promise you will see the fruit of your labor.

When people tell me they have been diagnosed, the most important factor they need to know is, if you are walking in the light Jesus shines on your pathway, you will make sound decisions. Psalm 18:28 (Amp) – *"For you cause my lamp to be lighted and to shine, the Lord my God illumines my darkness."*

As Dr. Caroline Leaf, author of *Who Switched off My Brain*, says 98 percent of all disease comes from thoughts. Alex Lloyd, developer of *The Healing Codes* agrees. Everyone has genes that lie dormant until a thought activates them. I absolutely despise genetic testing. But medical society is convincing women everywhere to be proactive to the possibility of genetics causing breast cancer. Women are making foolish decisions to butcher their bodies for no reason at all. They have allowed a doctor to plant a seed of concern into their minds, producing a harvest of fear.

Removing your breast does not guarantee that you will not get cancer in other parts of your body. Your breasts didn't cause the disease in the first place. People who go the conventional way rarely change their poor lifestyles. They think the doctors did the work for them, and they fail to discover the real root of the problem.

I met a woman at lunch the other day at my favorite raw restaurant. She was wearing a Susan G. Komen shirt. I asked her "Did you have breast cancer?" She softly replied, "I did." I told her that I too had breast cancer and that I was in the process of writing a book about how I chose to take the natural route. She told me that they scared her so bad, she went the conventional route and is still having a difficult time getting over the removal of her breasts. She asked me if the feelings she had were normal. And I said, "Of course they are."

When men are diagnosed with testicular cancer I am sure they think about it a little while before they give up a testicle. Yet women immediately give up their breasts without thinking about it first because somebody told them that their breasts weren't important.

Our breasts are very important parts of our sensuality. They keep our sweaters looking good, they are great weather girls, and you can nurse children with them. Breasts are a significant part of our bodies! The woman continued to share her story telling me that she is now in the process of undergoing additional reconstructive surgery—which they keep messing up.

People do not understand that doctors know surgery, chemo, and radiation are not the cure for cancer. They are still saying one day there will be a cure. After fifty-five years the conventional method of treatment only has a 5 percent survival rate. The only thing they have improved on is the hospitals are nicer, the breast reconstructive surgery is better and they've added some drugs to prevent you from getting so sick during chemo treatments. Chemo is chemo is chemo. Bottom line!

I realize that everybody has to make their own choice. But the main point I want you to walk away with from my book is not to make a decision in fear. Get educated. I have never felt healthier than I do now, and I feel so much younger, even though I am getting older. I sleep well, have healthy appetite, and love life!

Faith has been my most valuable commodity. It has carried me through the difficult times. God is faithful and He always comes through. I like to say that He's an 11:59 God and will show up on His time, not mine. I knew all along that I was going to be fine, and I am so thankful that He showed me in the beginning through a dream that I would be healed before going for a second opinion to the Disneyland of cancer facilities.

Even though I knew this, what would I choose to believe during my adventure at the Disneyland cancer center? Would I put my trust in the doctor's report or what God had shown me in a dream? Would I believe God's word that healing is one of His benefits and that the work was done at the cross? Or would I believe a piece of paper? Through all the difficult moments I faced, I chose to have blind faith. Though I could not yet see my healing, I trusted God to fulfill His promise to me.

One day I was walking Iggy and saw a lady wearing a beautiful platinum ribbon that represented cancer. Now let me be clear, you will never see me wearing anything that supports conventional cancer treatment and has fear attached to it. I will stand with my sisters, every one of them and support all along the way. But, no thank you, absolutely no badge for me.

I asked her, "Did you have cancer?" She said, "Yes, I had colon cancer." When I tell people I went the natural route they look at me horrified. I can't quite understand the look in their eyes when I tell them what I chose to do. Either I am plain crazy, or I am lying. This lady said to me that she never knew there were any other alternatives available to her. Doctors do not feel comfortable telling you the other routes you can take. Cancer is big business in the medical world. Hear me when I say, it is big business.

One day I do plan to design a necklace that will represent a nonprofit organization, which I will start. It will have a charm on it that says, "healed." Not survivor, not victim, not cut, poisoned or burned, but HEALED. When you go the natural route you don't have to survive surgery, chemo, or radiation. The only thing I had to get through was some lifestyle changes and some much needed detox. Nor will you have to survive a near death experience because you are not poisoning your body. The natural route builds the body versus breaking it down. I am not a survivor; I am healed and restored by my Father in Heaven.

If we were honest with ourselves we would admit that we constantly eat poorly, consuming way too much fast food, drink contaminated water, go to the doctor too much, and take too many antibiotics and over-the-counter medication. The human body is a survival machine that can heal itself if given the right tools. I believe those "right tools" address both the physical and emotional parts of our being. I know people who have eaten perfectly every single day of their life, yet they were never healed. They failed to enjoy life, be grateful, and have fun. What caused them to get cancer and never heal? What was so deep down in their soul that broke their bodies down?

What people have to realize is that you have to get to the root of what caused the cancer or disease. There are physical and emotional traumas attached to disease that we stuff down and don't take the time to deal with. Cutting your breast off will not fix these issues. You must take responsibility for finding the root cause and deal with the cellular memory.

Women are the worst, walking around pretending that everything is ok. Then there is the other side of the population, who are full of bitterness all the time. It's one extreme or the other.

I recently spoke to a lady who works in the home health care industry. She dreads more than anything when she has to work with older women because 95 percent of them are mean, hateful, grumpy, and ungrateful. They are old and upset because they didn't live their life to its fullest or life didn't turn out the way they expected it to. We all have these high and sometimes false expectations about life.

I thought by now I would be married, have kids, living in my dream home, and even have grandchildren. I had all these dreams and plans for myself, but none of them have happened yet. Life is to be fully lived. That's why I love animals so much. They live only in the now, they don't think about tomorrow. Maybe, that's why they are so loving and happy all the time.

We tend to be disappointed a lot of the time, about how our lives turned out. Was I happy when I was diagnosed with cancer? Absolutely not. Was that the plan I had for my life? No. Was it God's plan for my life? Of course not. But when I was diagnosed I had to make a choice, was I going to be happy or bitter? I came to a quick conclusion that we are all on borrowed time. You never know when your time is going to end. We think if we look healthy, eat well, and exercise we're going to live forever. But tomorrow, we could get hit by a car. We are all on borrowed time, and we have the choice to determine how we will live each day. I am going to live mine to the fullest!

I never once said, "Why me?" I did talk to God about my diagnosis and said, "If this is what has happened to me, then let's make the best of it." Yes, I needed to know why I got the disease, but not why me. The one thing I have learned from this is that life is short and I better enjoy every single minute of it. I plan on being here until a ripe old age.

Unhappiness and bitterness are wasted feelings, just like guilt, anger, and jealousy. Even though we are human and we will experience all of these emotions in a lifetime, it benefits us to get over them faster. God wants us to dwell and think on the beautiful things that happen in life. *Philippians 4:8 (NIV) – "Finally, brothers, whatever is true, whatever is noble, whatever is right, whatever is pure, whatever is lovely, whatever is admirable—if anything is excellent or praiseworthy—think about such things."*

I believe that breast cancer is also an issue of the heart. Most women I have interviewed during this time have told me they believe they got breast cancer because of the excessive stress in their lives or from a bad relationship. I also found that some women were diagnosed in the midst of a divorce when their hearts were broken. As I continued to dig deeper, there were women who suffered from being abused physically, mentally, and emotionally in their past, including myself.

In one of my favorite books, *The Healing Code*, it talks about breast cancer being an issue of trust and patience. If the person whom you love and trust the most violates you, a breaking of the trust occurs from that violation. This leaves the heart broken in many pieces and void of understanding. People, if you have a child that has been abused, you must address the issue immediately. No one took care of me when I was abused, and I believe that broken heartedness never healed leaving me to stuff it deep down inside.

Satan likes our secrets to remain hidden because if we stuff it down, the end result produces unhealthy emotions, reactions, and sickness. You've heard the old saying, "You're full of crap."

Well, it's true and that's not just physically, but emotionally too. If you knot up, everything inside you knots up.

If you don't deal with what really caused the disease, I believe that it can reoccur. Regardless of the route you take, you can juice all you want, take supplements, detox and even allow a doctor to cut and poison you. None of these things deal with the root of the disease. Deal with the issues of the heart.

My life has changed so much since the day I was diagnosed. I am grateful for the blessing it has turned out to be. It has made me look at things so differently. I have met so many wonderful people along the way, from doctors to researchers and all of them have played such an integral part in my journey. I can see my purpose so clearly now.

Being diagnosed allowed me to mend my ways and forgive my parents. It was learning and walking through the process of forgiveness that has allowed me to heal. If bad things have happened to you in your life, I want you to know that God can take those things and turn them into something beautiful. *Isaiah 61: 2-4 (NIV) – "…to comfort all who mourn, and provide for those who grieve in Zion – to bestow on them a crown of beauty instead of ashes, the oil of joy instead of mourning, and a garment of praise instead of a spirit of despair."*

I consistently speak life over myself and say I am healed. After two years, people still ask me, "How is your health Venus?" My reply is, "I am healed, and my health is perfect. How about yours?" You have to claim and know that you are healed. This disease will never afflict me again, not in one year or even five years down the road. Conventional patients have that five-year window hanging over their heads, which to me is five years of fear. The doctor knows that there is a significant chance of reoccurrence within the first five years.

Blind faith is like sowing a seed. The farmer cannot see the harvest with his eyes that lies in that tiny seed, yet he knows that if he waits patiently, the day will come when he will receive a beautiful harvest. I challenge you to do the same thing with your faith. Sow a tiny seed of trust in God and watch to see the results that will bloom right before your eyes.

Blind faith has taught me to say it was over when I was diagnosed, I just didn't realize it. The debt was paid at the cross. *I Peter 2:24 (MSG) – This is the kind of life you've been invited into, the kind of life Christ lived. He suffered everything that came his way so you would know that it could be done, and also know how to do it, step, by step.*

The magic pill for your disease is to walk in blind faith.

- Venus DeMarco

The Disneyland of Cancer Treatment Centers

May 2009 *It's a Monday morning, my car is packed, and I am off to get a second opinion. I will be staying with a friend's mom, Virginia, who is a wonderful Christian woman living in Houston. As I get closer to her home, my car begins to act funny. How can this be? My car is less than a year old. I get a block from Virginia's home when my steering wheel column locks up, and I realize that all the power steering fluid has leaked out. As the tears began to stream down my face and my body tenses with stress, I realize that the test of faith has begun.*

Obviously, I was a bit rattled by the time I arrived at Virginia's home. But as soon as I walked through her doors I remember feeling a peace that lingered in the air. It quickly soothed my weary heart. After settling in, I made a quick call to Lisa, my prayer partner at Shoreline, to share a dream I had had the night before.

In my dream, a lightening bolt struck my breast. I was awakened by the brightness of the light in my room as though it was really real. It didn't scare me nor did I think much about what had happened, I just peacefully drifted back to sleep. Lisa said she would look up the meaning in a dream book she had and get back to me. But we both knew without even checking that I had a visitation from God that night, and He was showing me that I was healed.

Lisa phoned me later to confirm that lightening means sudden miracle. How amazing that God would give me confirmation in a dream prior to everything I was about to go through and tell me that I was healed. Even though the test that I was about to have would not say I was healed. Blind faith is what has sustained me. Sometimes the miracle is done, but you don't know it because you can't see it. What you see isn't the truth. From that night on, I vowed to be steadfast in my faith, trusting God that I was healed even though I couldn't see the results.

When morning came and it was time to get ready for my appointment, Virginia was preparing to leave for work. I said, "I can't go alone, and besides I can't drive my car. Please go with me." Virginia was so gracious. She made a quick call into work and rearranged her day in order to take me to my appointment.

As we entered through the doors of the facility in Texas that I call the Disneyland of cancer, we were greeted by the reeking smell of sickness. Though the facility was elaborately decorated, I found it to be a very demonic, infested place. The first series of appointments would take me to a floor where

I would have my blood work and x-rays done. On display for our viewing pleasure was a lovely baby grand piano in the waiting room area. Soothing worship music would have helped to change the mood and atmosphere of this very dark place.

I really had no idea what was in store for me in the next few days. I literally gained ten pounds overnight due to the overwhelming stress I was feeling about my visit to the "theme park." I would find myself being thoroughly interrogated by a nurse from the questionnaire I had completed before going into the examination room. She wanted to know why I was taking a supplement called Turmeric. I told her I wanted to protect myself from all the radiation that they were going to expose me to during my visit. She smugly replied and said, "Nutrition doesn't work." I looked at her and told her maybe she should try it. Remember, I am a feisty, Italian girl who is not a push over when it comes to opinions.

They sent me off to meet with the oncologist, who was a very kind man. I begin to share with him the changes I had made in my diet. He said he understood why I felt so healthy because my blood work looked so good. I just wasn't healthy in my breast. I said to the oncologist, "Then I am not healthy somewhere else in my body, because my breasts didn't cause this. My poor breasts are developing an inferiority complex from all these accusations."

He asked me a series of questions about my family history. He wanted to know if anyone else in my family had ever had breast cancer. Yes, my grandmother on my mom's side and two aunts. I knew he was going to say that my breast cancer was genetic. However, I completely disagreed with him. I believe that their breast cancer came from an unhealthy lifestyle that they lived. Heavy drinking, eating the southern fried diet accompanied with a large dose of emotional stress is no prescription for healthy. At one point, my Grandmother remarried and chose to give up her kids. I am certain that this decision was one of regret, leaving my Grandmother filled with intense guilt and sadness. Besides, tell me why breast cancer is an epidemic now. What about 100 years ago? You never heard the term genetic because it just wasn't happening—nor was it happening with me. In my opinion, this diagnosis was not the result of genetics.

From the blood test results, the oncologist decided to cancel the CAT scan. Thank God! Do you know how much radiation is in a CAT scan? I would prefer to not do a Cat scan because of the radiation. I would consider a MRI.

Surveys have suggested that many CAT Scans are requested unnecessarily. Although, CAT Scans come with an additional risk of cancer (it can be estimated that the radiation exposure from a full body scan is the same as standing 2.4 km away from the World War II atomic bomb blasts in Japan.) (Information from Wikipedia) Now that should change anyone's mind.

Typical scan doses: (Note: A rem is a large dose of radiation, so the millirem (mrem), which is one thousandth of a rem, is often used for the dosages commonly encountered, such as the amount of radiation received from medical x-rays. An acute whole-body dose of less than 50 rem is typically subclinical and will produce nothing other than blood changes. Amounts from 50 to 200 rem may cause illness but will rarely be fatal. Doses of 200 to 1,000 rem will probably cause serious illness with poor outlook at the upper end of the range. Doses of more than 1,000 rems are almost invariably fatal.) In other words, a mammogram is equivalent to 1000 chest x-rays.

However, I was willing to let them do just about anything to me that day in order to confirm that the first doctor's diagnosis was accurate. I remember the strange look the doctor gave me when the nurse left the room, and I said, "Don't look at me like I'm crazy." He replied, "I don't think you are crazy at all."

My day at the amusement park for cancer finally came to a close and boy was I ready to call it a day. Virginia and I drove back to her home to relax for the remainder of the evening.

May 2009 *Morning came quickly, and I am headed back to the "Cancerland" to have the mammogram done. Mark my words, I WILL NEVER HAVE ANOTHER MAMMOGRAM AGAIN!!! They are extremely dangerous, with concentrated amounts of radiation being shot into your breast as they are compressed and flattened like pancakes between two metal plates. This procedure can damage the lymph system and aggravate the tumor, releasing cancerous cells throughout the entire body.*

As soon as I walk into the room I am greeted by the technician who says, "I was just praying for you before you arrived." I have never been squeezed, pressed, or turned in so many directions. I ask the technician if she has ever heard of miracles happening here. She replies, "Once there was a rumor that someone who supposedly had cancer returned for another test and the results showed no signs of the disease." She pauses. "You never have to do anything you don't want to do." Kind of odd...

After I was done with the mammogram, I was sent off to get an ultra sound. They had me wait in a strange little dressing room area with a curtain. As I sat there waiting and waiting for over an hour, I began to see employees leave for the day. At that point the lady who had done my mammogram walked by, and I remember complaining to her how long I had been sitting there. She never turned her body toward me, only her head. "Remember, you don't have to do anything you don't want to do."

I finally got into the ultrasound room, where to my surprise I had to wait another half hour. When the technician did come in, she immediately engaged in conversation with me about her son living in Austin. He worked at some juice bar. She said he was "all into health and thinks that juicing and stuffs works."

I said, "It really does work." I find it a bit surprising that doctors don't believe in the power of proper nutrition.

As she started to do the ultra sound, things began to get very eerie. The radiologist came into the exam room, which happened to be one of the darkest ultrasounds rooms I had ever been in. It was completely dark except for the light from the machine. I felt such a demonic presence.

The radiologist told me some of the cells had spread from the first biopsy. Followed by the fact that she would like to do a very aggressive biopsy today to determine what type of cancer it is. I replied, "My doctor didn't prescribe that." She said it didn't matter.

I knew that if I let them do the aggressive biopsy it could metastasize the cancer right then and there. It doesn't matter what kind of cancer you have or if you are stage 1 or stage 4. Cancer is cancer is cancer. Metastasizing cancer is what kills people.

Then, clear as day, I heard a voice say, "Get up now, put your clothes on, and get out of there."

I wiped the gel off my breasts and left immediately.

When I got out into the hallway it was completely dark, and no one was left on floor. I looked at my phone and saw that Virginia had texted me, "Something is really wrong. Get out of there now." I rushed out as quickly as I could and jumped into the car. I was pretty freaked at that point and asked Virginia if she would take me to Lakewood Church since I had been reading Dodie Osteen's book, *Healed of Cancer*.

As we walked through the doors of the church we were greeted by the security guard who told us we could walk around but asked us not to go into the sanctuary. He didn't want us in the sanctuary due to liability purposes and the dangers of not having all the lights on in the building. Like a little kid, guess where I went? Straight to the sanctuary.

As we were sitting there praying, a girl appeared out of the blue. I found her behavior to be extremely odd. She kept saying that Jesus was the lamb. She had a very big head and shared with us that she had an out of body experience the last time she was here. I looked at Virginia and said, "That's it. I have had enough. Let's get out of here."

Once we got outside, we both asked, "Where in the world did she come from?" Neither of us saw her enter the sanctuary.

Satan was having me followed.

Though the day was absolutely crazy, I was able to experience what other women go through when they are desperately seeking answers for the diagnosis of breast cancer. You would not see me enter through the gates at the Disneyland of cancer ever again! I was committed to researching every avenue I could to heal God's natural way.

May 2009 *My journey has come to an end here, and I am ready to go home. As I sit waiting for my car to be fixed, I realize that I have to take some time off of work and de-stress so that my heart rate will go back down. Pondering my next move, my sister calls. She tells me that the doctor from the treatment center is on the phone and is worried about me. Gee whiz, now they're tracking me down through my family.*

I call the doctor back. "Venus, what are you going to do," he asks. I say I am heading to Myrtle Beach to see Dr. Cotter, who specializes in oxygen treatments; I am going to heal by God's natural route.

He is freaked out but he knows he can't tell me what to do. So, instead he asks that I call him and keep him posted on how things are going. I take down his cell phone number.

As I sit here today writing this book, I am looking at that number written on the back of his business card—I think instead of a call, I will just send him a copy of my book. I still receive letters to date from the cancer treatment center asking if I am cancer free. What a crock! All they really wanted was every penny they could get from my insurance company and they succeeded!

After all the new inventions in modern medicine, many physicians' study results show the success rate for the conventional method of treating breast cancer is still only 5 percent after all these years. Why would I choose 5 percent when I can choose 90 percent success rate by going God's natural way? I have worked in the skincare business for over thirty years and we were taught the importance of good nutrition. Knowing what I know about the human body, it's easy for me to choose God's way. I can't imagine burning my body with radiation, cutting my body parts off, or poisoning myself. I know that this will take a lot of work and faith but I am going to trust God to direct me on this journey to get healthy.

The first thing to remember during the journey is that God

is still working behind the scenes regardless of what is seen or felt. I am healed!

When a brave person takes a stand, the spines of others are stiffened.

- Billy Graham

Redneck Riviera

May 2009 *Right now my emotions are well intact, and I am feeling pretty upbeat considering all I have been through. I am preparing for the next leg of my journey as I continue to gather more knowledge about God's natural way to heal.*

I know that I need to meet Dr. Cotter, but my finances are extremely tight. I am concerned about meeting all my obligations. But thanks to an anonymous individual who so generously paid my rent, I now can go on this trip.

Whoever you are and if you are reading this book, thank you from the bottom of my heart for your gift. You have been a very important part of my journey and your gift was one of many miracles that I have received.

Continued *I love my sister very much but I needed her support right now more than she can ever imagine. I have been calling her over and over again, even trying to bribe her into meeting* *me in Myrtle Beach, which is much closer to where she lives than Austin.*

I was just diagnosed with breast cancer a little over a month ago, and no one from my family has to come to see me yet. I am so frustrated with them that I even called my aunt to tell her how hurt I was and that I hated my family. (I don't really hate my family - I just hate their lack of support during this time.)

I felt like it shouldn't have taken so much convincing for my sister to come support me. She should have said. "You're going to be in Myrtle Beach? That's no problem. I will be there.

Tuesday, May 26, 2009 *I am leaving on a jet plane headed to Myrtle Beach, better known as the Redneck Riviera to meet Dr. Cotter for the very first time and to hang out with my sister. I have no idea what to expect on this trip, but I am praying to get great results from oxygen bath treatments and to gather important information that will help me to heal.*

In case I have your curiosity stirred, it's called Redneck Riviera because it's one of the most affordable places to go in the good old south.

As for Dr. H. Thomas Cotter, well he is the recipient of many awards and is world-renowned for his pioneering work in the realm of homeopathic treatment and eradication of many devastating global ailments. He has over thirty years of experience and has dedicated much of his efforts to research. Dr. Cotter partnered with an anonymous chemist/inventor to discover perhaps the most significant breakthrough in Medical History… Liquid Prana.

One of my main reasons for wanting to meet Dr. Cotter is to find out more about his oxygen treatment baths and how they work. Research shows that cancer cannot survive in an oxygenated environment because it's an anaerobic cell. These cells like a very acidic and non-oxygenated environment.

The bath treatments Dr. Cotter developed quickly invade the body with oxygen, and I firmly believe this is what will keep the cancer from spreading throughout my body.

I was proactive in my healing from the very beginning.

Later that day *"Santa" greeted me when I arrived today. I sure hope he brings me good health and wellbeing for Christmas this year! We came back to a beautiful home that is located on the beach and is owned by a man named Mark Johnson, who is being treated by Old St. Nick as well. Mark has generously allowed a few of Dr. Cotter's (who is from California) patients to stay there during treatments.*

Now that I'm settled I've been given a glass of Liquid Prana Water while I wait for my turn to take an oxygen treatment bath. Liquid Prana is the first and only water of its kind. After enrichment with a proprietary technology, the water is super-oxygenated. When consumed, this water replenishes the body by enriching the cells with oxygen. This allows the cells to repair themselves, thus making their host healthier and more energized.

This water is unbelievable! I can't get enough of it! I just keep drinking and drinking it even though I am not really that thirsty. But my body keeps saying I want more. It's very obvious that I needed the life source that was contained in this water.

My bath is ready. I jump right in to the large tub without checking the temperature of the water. It is so hot, that I immediately hop out. Someone to come help me... This man who had been diagnosed with prostrate cancer is sitting on the couch. He is so kind to come to my rescue and adjust the temperature perfectly for me.

After that first bath treatment, I realized I hadn't been that calm and relaxed in a long time. I could already see my stress level going down. After a long day, I climbed into bed and drifted off to sleep very quickly. I slept like a baby that night—twelve solid hours. By the way, rest is vital to your healing. The body repairs itself while you are sleeping. Be sure to get enough zzz's.

Wednesday, May 27, 2009 *I'm starting to enjoy these baths. It's taken a while to get used to the regimen of what I am required to do. Sitting still for a solid hour isn't that easy in our fast-paced society. As I learn how to enjoy being still and to relax during these bath treatments, I read and meditate on the 40 healing scriptures from Dodie Osteen's book "Healed of Cancer." This helps me purify my mind and be reminded of God's faithfulness. We are made up of mind, body, and soul. Healing needs to happen in all three of these areas when you are diagnosed with an illness.*

Tonight is dinner with the boys! Cotter is whipping up a yummy batch of curry chicken with his handsome sidekick Chef Mark. What a warm and friendly place this has turned out to be. Everyone here came to be healed, yet unselfishly is willing to help one another in the time of need. What a beautiful picture of grace being extended.

Thursday would prove to be a very difficult morning for me. I cried a lot during my bath treatment that day. I know it was a much-needed cry. It is so easy to bottle up your feelings and just put on a happy face for everyone else. But there's nothing like a good cry to help flush out and rid you of any negative emotions. There have been studies done that show once you stop crying your body will move into a state of relaxation and your breathing and heart rate will return to normal as well.

Thursday, May 28, 2009 Today, I met an amazing twelve-year-old girl who has such incredible insight and strength for her age. Her father was diagnosed with stage 4 colon and liver cancer. He had surgery to remove parts of his colon but chose note to have chemotherapy treatments. There is less cancer now, but he still has three tumors left in his liver. She comes here with her mother so that her dad can get the oxygen bath treatments three times a day.

I asked how they found Dr. Cotter and she said that her dad was talking to a man named Ray at church about what was going on with his health and how he didn't know what to do. Ray told him about Mark's story and contacted him to see if he would open up his home.

Within approximately two months of the treatments, Dr. Cotter *has witnessed healing taking place in her dad's body. When he first arrived he had a lot of moles on his back that are now practically smooth, and his face is clear.*

Before he started taking the bath treatments he didn't have much energy. Just recently he spent an entire day with daughter, watched her play tennis, then went to the movies and hung out some more. He is able to enjoy doing things again.

Later *I'm start to see the signs that my body is beginning to detoxify. My tonsils are swollen and my lymphatic system is moving stuff out. You know what they say, better out than in.*

I call the Disneyland of cancer treatment centers to request them to fax my test results over to Dr. Cotter so he can review them and share his recommendations for healing.

I never did hear back from the center. I think they may have been upset since they didn't receive any more insurance money from me and my Ta Tas.

That night Thank God that Ms. Bonnie brought us dinner tonight because these men eat like crap. They only cook one good meal a day, then the rest of the day they eat junk. Remember to do what your mom always taught you and eat your veggies. Nutrition is such a key factor in healing.

Vern's wife—the twelve-year-old girl's mother—shared with me that they lost their second son in a car wreck. I can't imagine how difficult that must be for a parent to lose a child nor how they learn to cope and try to move on after such a tragedy. They both have a personal relationship with the Lord that I am sure has helped them deal with their grief and has given them strength during Vern's health issues.

Vern's brother is actually a Pastor; no doubt they look to him for spiritual reinforcement as well as encouragement. Like most people who come into the home they know that all things are possible with God. Matthew 19:26 (NIV) – "Jesus looked at them and said, "With man this is impossible, but with God all things are possible." I don't know how people manage in everyday life or in a crisis without God. He gives me hope!

Friday, May 29, 2009 *I can't believe it is Friday already! The week has just flown by. This morning I enjoyed a cup of coffee with Dr. Cotter as we overlooked the ocean, and I can say it doesn't get much better than this. During my bath this morning, I read Dodie Osteen's book again. It always seems to help remind me of God's promises. Controlling your thought pattern during this time is crucial. You have to get rid of the fear that will try to inundate your mind. 2 Timothy 1:7 – "For God did not give us a spirit of fear…"*

In other news, my sister is coming today, and I can't wait to see her. She has not seen me since I was diagnosed. Of course, of all days today I am starting not to feel so well due to my body detoxing. Instead of staying at the house with the boys, we will be staying at a beautiful ocean view hotel while she is here. I must say things are lot less expensive in the Redneck Riviera—ocean view suite, $140 a night.

After we checked in, we headed to the beach for some rest and relaxation. I love the smell of the ocean air, the sound of the waves rolling in, and the sand between my toes. I also love a little drama from time to time. I have to warn you, I still hadn't given up the cocktails at that time, and I probably had one too many that particular afternoon.

Later that day *My sister and I are visiting a little cozy beach bar to grab a couple of drinks. There is a group of good old southern boys to our left that appear to be quite entertaining—and handsome. How can they resist two hot flirty Italian chicks like me and sis?*

I hear myself laughing a lot during our conversations with them. I just love to laugh and have fun. Besides, laughter is such good medicine. It helps to reduce your stress level and improves your mood. At this point, I can say I am in a very good mood!

One of the guys hands me his business card, and as I looked it over I notice his name is T.K. Brown. I'm quite curious what T.K. stands for. Rather than ask, I name him Titty Kent Brown—which I announce to the entire bar. His friends are cracking up, and so am I.

I must say I've always enjoyed a good laugh, even at myself. I told you this was a journey. I am sure that to this day, Titty Kent Brown is being harassed by his friends.

After our fun time with the boys, we headed back to the house so I could take my oxygen treatment bath. But, by the time I returned to the hotel I had started running a fever with really bad chills. My sister was worried and upset, but Dr. Cotter said not to worry.

At some point that night during a conversation with my sister, I recall telling her I didn't want to die over and over again. She continued to reassure me that I wasn't going to die. I am five years older than my younger sister, and I can't tell you how grateful I was that she was by my side that night. There was a lot of mucus coming out of my body, and the chills were so extreme that my sister had to keep getting up and putting more blankets on me throughout the night.

Dr. Cotter again reassured my sister and I the next day, explaining that I was going through a detoxification process. He said all the symptoms I had were completely normal. He explained that this has nothing to do with my breasts. This was my body getting rid of the junk so that I could heal. The treatments were causing my body to detox, which was essential in my healing process. Everyone in the house was getting great results from the oxygen baths including me.

Sunday, May 31, 2009 *I am taking my bath, and I am completely burnt out at this point. I know that I am leaving tomrrow, and my emotions are running on high. I am in the tub crying. What am I doing here? Am I crazy?*

I hear the Lord, "I told you I have already taken care of it. You are OK, get on with it, have fun with your sister tonight. I've already take care of it."

What timing and affirmation to hear directly from God and that He would remind me again, that He took care of my disease way back on the cross. My family may not have been here all along but my Father in Heaven is here every step of the way. I feel so loved by Him! Words cannot describe the peace that I feel right now.

I can't wait to share my experience with Mark. During my story, and right in front of his 22-year-old son, he asks if I had an orgasm. I can't believe that he just said that. He just got back from church, and right in front of his son? I guess it just goes to show that men have a one-track mind.

During the days at the Redneck Riviera, I would spend time with my sister hanging out and enjoying the beach. In the evenings we would stop by the house for me to take my bath treatments, visit with the other guests, and on occasion help clean up after those messy men.

At the end of our time there, my sister and I stopped by the house to say our goodbyes. This was extremely difficult for me to do since we had all grown so close in such a short period of time. I got to live with four men for a week, each of which was so kind and loving. That trip was truly such a great experience for me.

Tuesday, June 1, 2009 *I drove my sister to the airport this morning. I can't tell you how much I enjoyed my time with her. I am beginning to feel somewhat emotional as she leaves.*

Now I'm back in the hotel room, and I am so aware of how lonely I feel. I wonder if I will have a hard time trying to board the plane with the flu-like symptoms I am experiencing from this detox process. Everyone is already freaked out because of the swine flu epidemic. There are even signs at the airport that read: "If you have flu-like symptoms do not board the plane." But I don't have the flu; I am just in a state of detox. Of course, if you tell people you are detoxing, they will think you just got out of rehab.

I'm calling my friend Elaine before trying to board the plane to ask her if my symptoms are normal. She reassures me that they are.

Even after arriving home, it took me a solid week to completely detox and start to feel better. The first round of detox was pretty intense. But thank God every physical detox since has been a lot easier with the exception of an emotional detox, which is a whole other story.

My time and adventure at the Redneck Riviera has come to an end for now. I am so thankful to my sister who was there for me when I really needed her. As for all the men at the house they were kind, caring, and respectful to me. They gave me a sense of security and forever impacted my life. My hats off to the good ole southern boys who made me laugh—even you Titty Kent Brown.

I wouldn't trade what I learned on this trip—including the detoxification process I had to go through to begin my healing process. I felt so blessed, and I knew I was moving in the right direction.

"The road of life twists and turns and no two directions are ever the same. Yet our lessons come from the journey, not the destination."

By Don Williams, Jr.

Mexico or Bust

June 2009 *It has been a few months since I was diagnosed with breast cancer. I am eating right, taking the correct supplements, plus downing my daily shots of wheatgrass and poopin' like a big dog. That's what happens when you are drinking Green Smoothies and eating a veggie based diet. Lots of fiber keeps you extremely regular, if you know what I mean. I am consistently doing my T-Tapp workouts to improve my lymphatic system and walking a lot. I am feeling good about the things that I am doing to take care of myself now.*

Thank God for my dog. He will not allow me to lock myself away from the rest of the world. He makes me take him for daily walks, which allows me to take in some good fresh air and a little sunshine. I want all the Vitamin D I can get.

There are a couple of things bugging me right now. Number one on the list are my hormones. They are completely out of whack! I am having a difficult time sleeping because the night sweats are completely out of control. I'm also having continuous hot flashes all day. This sucks! It's a red flag and big concern for me. The other thing I am struggling with is my emotions. I haven't gotten to the point of fully grasping that my body will heal itself, which leaves an avenue for fear to creep in at times. I am also exploring every possible piece of information I can get my hands on that may help me heal.

I remember right around this time there was one day at work when I was giving one of my clients a facial and sharing some of my story. She said to me, "Oh my gosh! My best friend's father is a holistic doctor, who specializes in natural cures for cancer." Isn't that amazing how God can put the right person at the right time in your path? The information she shared with me was extremely relevant for my journey and would prove to be a valuable piece that would help complete the puzzle of my story.

I immediately contacted Dr. Hines' office and scheduled my first appointment with him. He has two office locations—one in San Angelo, plus another clinic called Hope Wellness Center in Acuna, Mexico that he shares with two other doctors. I will be meeting him in Del Rio because the natural treatments they do for cancer are not allowed into U.S. Their patients gather to meet them in this border town, and then they travel across together to the clinic.

I have never been to this part of Texas before, so I contact a friend of mine, Kate Fly, who is a native Texan that was not working at the time. She agreed to join me on this trip and was even willing to drive. That in itself was a Godsend, since I, at that point, didn't have the energy to drive for long periods of time or handle a lot of stress. Even the simplest things tended to overwhelm me, and my goal was to minimize anything that would cause unhealthy stress.

July 4 Weekend 2009 *On the road again, can't wait to get on the road again… It's Mexico or bust. We left for Del Rio the Sunday after the Fourth of July. During the drive, Kate told me about this healer in Austin that she volunteers with twice a week. She recommends that I check him out. My initial reaction is surprisingly hesitantcy in contacting him because of my beliefs. But, I take his information and consider touching base with him when we return to Austin. I am very open to discovering the truth and willing to consider meeting with anyone I feel may be helpful to me and my Ta Tas.*

Del Rio was a very friendly border town with a lot of good Mexican food. After checking into our hotel room we decided to check out the town and our options for dinner—Mexican or fast food. Neither of these was well suited for my special diet at the time. However, instead of feeling guilty over food, which to me is worse than not eating something that's in your diet, I made the best choice I could with the available options.

July 2009 *As the sun rises to kiss the morning with its beautiful rays, I wait with anticipation to see what the day holds for me and my bodacious Ta Tas. I have no idea what to expect from my appointment or what Dr. Hines. I don't even know what he looks like.*

I see a tall and handsome man who has a voice like Rick Bayless. If you don't know who Rick Bayless is, he is an amazing TV chef with a show called Mexico One Plate at a Time. Wouldn't you know that as soon as I hear his voice, I immediately started craving Mexican food? Muy Bueno!

Even now, when I speak with Dr. Hines on the phone, I get an intense craving for Mexican.

The other patients had also gathered at the restaurant for appointments with Dr. Hines and his colleagues loaded into a van to travel together into Acuna, Mexico. Kate and I followed them in our car. I remember how overwhelmingly poverty stricken the town was. However, the clinic, which is called Hope Wellness Center, was actually a very beautiful Mexican-style building located right next to an orphanage.

Later that day *This clinic is a place of hope, health, and healing. Hope has a unique approach to clinical medicine. Each patient is treated according to his or her individual concerns instead of receiving "cookie cutter" treatment for a particular ailment. Conventional medicine has given up on most of our patients, but the word "incurable" does not daunt the people of this clinic. They are not discouraged when some say, "No one has ever gotten well from this disease." The patients routinely recover from life-threatening or supposedly incurable diseases.*

Many people do not realize that diseases considered incurable in one country are often successfully treated in another. For example, Chinese doctors use intravenous garlic extract to successfully treat viral meningitis. German, Russian, and

Cuban doctors use intravenous ozone to kill viruses of all types. In England, homeopathic medicine is used in lieu of vaccinations, and is also used to treat psychological disorders. In Asia, acupuncture is sometimes used as the sole anesthetic during surgery. Having a global medical perspective is critical for those seeking the very best chance of recovery in my opinion. They adhere to that global perspective in the treatment of their patients at Hope.

Hope has no allegiance to any drug company, machine, or latest gadget. They keep an open mind—but also a scientific filter—to find the best treatments possible for their patients. Statements like, "My headache started right after I got some dental work done," or "Ever since I started on that high blood pressure medicine, I just can't sleep," are key truths they use to determine the root of the problem.

The core values at Hope Wellness Center are listening to the patients, diligently searching for the latest research on all ailments, and earnestly seeking to find and cure for the root of each patient's problem.

Some of the therapies they do include:

- Superior nutrition and supplementation (oral and IV)
- Magnetic therapy
- Oxygen therapy
- Ozone therapy

- Live cell therapy

- And an arsenal of various natural substances and when necessary conventional therapies.

Hope views diseases such as cancer, Parkinson, Lupus, heart failure, and Lyme as a whole body issue rather than an isolated problem. The breakdown of a person's immune system, poor nutrition, poor elimination, lack of restful sleep, chronic stress, toxicity build up, pathogen burdens, and a combination of all of the above result in more than your body can tolerate, and systems start breaking down. Their treatments work at a cellular level to rehabilitate damaged cells and turn them back into healthy cells. Some treatments are designed to eliminate pathogens such as parasites, viruses, yeast, fungus, and bacteria while others help cleanse and detoxify your body.

Later that day *I find Dr. Hines to be a very brilliant and passionate man. He lives his life to help people. As a former Pastor he knows the Bible very well and has a very compassionate bedside manner. He is so dedicated to helping people with their health that he has driven from San Angelo to the clinic in Mexico every week for the past fifteen years.*

Since 1994, Dr. Hines has served as the Director of Clinical Research at Hope Clinics International in Acuna, Mexico. The clinic specializes in the treatment of advanced degenerative diseases. In 2007, he established the Hormonal Balance Clinic of San Angelo, Texas where he utilizes nutrition, diet, and lifestyle management to normalize the function of the endocrine system. He just recently co-authored the book, *The Road to Health* with Laura Shroeder, which provides detailed and effective dietary strategies to restore normal gastrointestinal tract function, alleviate blood sugar deregulation, and chronic fatigue.

My appointment lasted for three solid hours. During that time Dr. Hines shared so much information with me that my brain was on overload. It was almost too much for me to take in and absorb. He also ran some blood tests and the results indicated that I had a fungus in my body. He said that most cancers are actually fungus related, which is why it's so important to be on natural anti-fungals like chaga mushrooms, wild oil of oregano, and Pau D' Arco tea. These are just some of the natural anti-funguls. Dr. Hines also prescribed some heavy duty anti-fungal supplements for me.

The main objective for going to see Dr. Hines was to gather some more information on the IV Treatments and any other natural options they offered for treating cancer. I was not aware on the front end how much time would be required for these treatments. After hearing the details plus the amazing success rate I knew I couldn't live in Del Rio at a hotel for six weeks. I made the decision that this was not the best option for me at the time. The big drawback for me is that I am single, an owner of a new business, and the bread winner of my household. There was not an option to close down my business and drag my dog Iggy with me to Del Rio to live in a hotel for six weeks.

The important thing I gained from my visit with Dr. Hines was that he discovered I had a fungus in my body—another missing piece of the puzzle. Dr. Hines had a wealth of information and will always be a part of my life forever. One suggestion he had for me was to find an Infrared sauna. I wasn't able to find one that I could use on a daily basis, so I started doing hot Yoga. It's not Bikrim, but I do it at a studio close to my home. Even though I have only seen him one time, I have stayed in contact with him and his lovely wife Sissy.

July 6, 2009 Kate and I are on the road again… this time back to Austin. During one of our conversations, she told me that her best friend's mom—whose name is Sunny Markham—developed this product called Pomegranate Breast Oil. The formula has medicinal qualities and capacity to fight abnormal cells in breast tissue. I love how again; God has put the right person at the right time on my path. This is just another piece I will add to the puzzle when I returned to Austin.

I learned a lot on this trip, but it's now time to say adios Mexico and hola Austin!

Proverbs 3:5&6 – "Trust in the Lord with all your heart and lean not on your own understanding; in all your ways submit to Him, and He will make your paths straight."

Home Sweet Home

July 2009 *Dorothy from the Wizard of Oz said it so well, "There is no place like home." Though I don't live in Kansas or own a pair of red sparkly shoes, I want to go home! Not only do I sleep better in my own bed, but I miss my sidekick, Iggy.*

During my visit with Dr. Hines in Mexico, not only did I learn about the specific treatments they have for cancer at their facility, but he imparted a wealth of knowledge. For instance, I received some very important information about fungus and how it can be misdiagnosed as cancer.

But, I just couldn't imagine living in Del Rio for six weeks and crossing the border into Mexico every single day for holistic treatments. I truly felt that it was better for me to return home after my visit. A very important part of the journey is determining what works best for you. And home was my best option.

July 2009 *Now that I am back in Austin, I find myself asking,* *what am I going to do? I know I have to keep moving forward and spend as much time as possible increasing my knowledge on the importance of consuming living foods. Keep in mind, it's only been few months since I was first diagnosed, but I am implementing significant changes in my diet that are crucial to my physical well being.*

I spent a lot of money on food, juicing, supplements, books, and CD'S. Plus I was trying to determine the right foods to eat and the proper supplementation to take. By the way, everybody has advice for you, and it will be up to you to weigh out the good from the bad.

One fun thing I did try was a raw food cooking class. Proper preparation of food is important, so that it maintains all the enzymes, micronutrients, and antioxidants. Most foods we consume are depleted of the nutrients that are so vital to our health. When you hear the term raw food, immediately most of us will say no thank you. That's why I took this class. It's important that you enjoy the food you eat in order for it to become a permanent part of your lifestyle. I now thoroughly enjoy preparing raw food meals for friends and myself. I am here to tell you, there are some delicious and filling raw food recipes that will surprise you and your family.

As I continued to review things that might be beneficial to my health, I recalled the information my friend Kate shared with me on our trip to Mexico. She had mentioned that her best friend's mom had successfully developed this product called Pomegranate Breast Oil, which was developed to promote

The Healing Journey of My Bodacious Ta Tas

breast health. The formula has medicinal qualities with a key ingredient called Ellagic acid, which has the capacity to fight abnormal cells along with, mustard seed to detox the breast tissue, and amber which opens up the heart chakra

I contacted Sunny Markham, who is the founder of "The Gathering for Health" headquartered in Austin, and shared with her who I was and how I got her information. She was so passionate about the product that she agreed to stop by my office to share in detail with me the benefits of this beautiful oil.

When she arrived at my office, we went into my facial room so that she could show me how to properly use the Pomegranate Breast Oil. We both took off our tops and she demonstrated for me on herself this beautiful type of breast massage that really helps to promote lymphatic flow. Isn't this just like every man's dream? Here are two women with their tops off, massaging their breast in a very specific way to stimulate lymphatic flow and detox the breast. I didn't think anything of it, and this wasn't sexy to us at all. Again, let me stress, I was exploring every natural healing source that was available to me.

The message I want everyone to get as they are reading this book is the importance of being proactive with your health, especially when it comes to preventing cancer. One of the ways of doing that is to massage the breast with this oil. The pomegranate oil rejuvenates the cells and the skin of the breast. I personally have incorporated this practice into my daily schedule and I believe that every woman should do the same.

While she was demonstrating the massage technique, I started to cry; because that was the first time I'd touched my breast since the diagnosis. Breast cancer is such an emotional journey with intense fear attached to it. I had blamed my breasts when they had nothing to do with this diagnosis. I had almost become obsessed with the tumor.

July 2009 *When I said I would try anything, good or bad, well I meant it. I scheduled an appointment to get a lymphatic massage. In case you are wondering exactly what that is, a lymphatic massage stimulates the lymph—a colorless fluid that travels through vessels in the lymphatic system and carries cells that help fight infection and disease. I explained to the female masseur that I had been diagnosed with breast cancer and she insisted on including a special treatment that would heal me. She held this lovely crystal over me and let it spin in circles. She said the crystal would draw the tumor out of my body. It's pretty amazing how many people think they can actually heal. I truly believe this woman's intentions were good, but I knew that a crystal was not going to heal me.*

Just a word of caution, be careful who you see and what you do. Don't become so desperate that fear causes you to make foolish decisions. I am very fortunate not to have been swept away by some of the people I've found and their practices. It's important to have a reliable sounding board. I try to keep my family and friends in the loop of what I am doing. A solid foundation is a must!

Each week I continue to invest more money, spend time researching and reading everything I can. I have also been inspired by listening to others share their stories. I ran across a lady who changed her diet to 100 percent raw food, no cooked foods whatsoever, no coffee, and was completely healed of breast cancer.

I know that I have made the right decision not to go the conventional route. By faith, yes by faith, I know that my tumor will be completely dissolved and I will be healthy and whole.

> **"Home is the one place in all this world where hearts are sure of each other. It is the place of confidence. It is the place where we tear off that mask of guarded and suspicious coldness which the world forces us to wear in self-defense, and where we pour out the unreserved communications of full and confiding hearts. It is the spot where expressions of tenderness gush out without any sensation of awkwardness and without any dread of ridicule."**
>
> **- Frederick W. Robertson**

A Year of Discovery

During that first year, I learned so many things about cancer, God, my faith, my emotions, my hormones, the importance of live food, and so much more. If I can stress one other very critical thing, don't become your disease. Learn how to enjoy life along the journey, even when it's difficult. Remember, God is always working behind the scenes even though you cannot see or feel Him, learn not to rush ahead of Him.

***August 2009** What a time of discovery this has been! I spent this year looking into good and bad options to treat breast cancer. I had mammograms, ultrasounds, blood tests, visited the Disneyland of cancer treatment centers, detoxed multiple times, experienced the benefits of oxygen bath treatments, crossed the border into Mexico, and learned that cancer is a biological process affecting the entire body. Cancer is not something that you can just cut, poison, or burn. Cancer has a switch. It can be turned on or off. I also discovered that fungus can be misdiagnosed as breast cancer, and that everyone wants to be a healer, and much, much more.*

The main thing is that without God, I could not have done any of this or even made it through the darkness. By His grace, He has upheld me. Isaiah 41:10 - "So do not fear, for I am with you; do not be dismayed, for I am your God. I will strengthen you and help you; I will uphold you with my righteous right hand."

The more you educate yourself, the more knowledge you will have in making wise decisions. I am constantly learning about supplementation, how to alkalize my body, reduce inflammation and kill cancer stem cells. Some of the things that I implemented into my daily routine during the first year were:

- God and prayer:

    Without God and faith, I wouldn't have made it this far. Take time to find a local church, where others can support you along the journey. Psalm 91: 14 – "Because he loves me," says the Lord, "I will rescue him; I will protect him, for he acknowledges my name. He will call on me, and I will answer him; I will be with him in trouble, I will deliver him and honor him and show him my salvation."

- Juicing fruits and vegetables:

    Juicing extracts all fiber (pulp) from foods, so when drinking the juice it is 100 percent free of pulp. When you juice, these juices become pre-digested, meaning they go into the bloodstream immediately by passing any need for digestion. It is in pure juice form. Absorbing 100 percent of the nutrients is why juicing is an incredible way to feed our bodies. I like to start my day off with a green juice, but remember you can drink green juices all day. When juicing, juice a lot of vegetables and little fruit. If you are sick, stick to just green juices to keep your sugar intake as low as possible.

- Follow a vegan diet:

  Follow a local, plant-based diet as much as possible. It's important to remove or heavily reduce the animal products in your diet. If you do choose to keep some animal products, keep it to a minimum and ensure they are completely organic, raised on sustainable farms, and certified humane. Local farms are always the best. Or, just make it easy. Try the vegetarian way of life and eat a plant-based diet.

- Daily shots of wheat grass:

  Not only will wheat grass boost your health, but it will detox the liver, purify the blood, and aid in keeping the colon clean.

- Green smoothies:

Green smoothies are when you blend your fruits and vegetables together in a high-speed blender, such as the VitaMix. All green leafy greens have cell walls mainly built of cellulose. These are very difficult for our bodies to break down to access the dense nutrition the greens supply. Since most people do not sit and chew their greens until they are juiced, blending the greens with the blender allows the machine to do most of the chewing. This makes the nutrients more accessible to the body. They will provide your body with the food it needs to heal itself. I know some of you might be saying, yuck I am not drinking anything green. Just try it. You will be pleasantly surprised!

- Natural supplementation:

   Supplementation is to stimulate your immune system and build the body back up, such as anti-inflammatory and antioxidant supplements plus other different herbs that are known to kill cancer stem cells and get rid of excessive bad estrogen in the body.

- Pomegranate breast oil:

   I added the lymphatic massage and oil twice daily,d which promotes breast health.

- Getting my hormones in balance:

    Hormones impact your body at the cellular level and your overall health depends on maintaining healthy cells. Get those hormones in check.

- Balanced my emotions:

    When the negative thoughts begin to race through your mind, take control of them and replace them with positive things. Reading scriptures, from Dodie Osteen's book, *Healed of Cancer,* helped me to start replacing the wrong thoughts with words of hope and healing.

    Remove as much stress from your life as possible. Keep short accounts with people and forgive quickly. If there is anything or anyone who is causing you extreme anxiety, I suggest taking a break from that environment until you are at a healthy state to address the situation better. Your health is a priority.

- Rest:

    Even God rested after the sixth day of creation. The body repairs itself while we sleep, which helps us to fight off sickness. It is crucial to get at least seven to nine hours of sleep a night.

- Exercise:

    It's a great thing to keep your body active, sweat, and move the lymphatic system.

I know that I have shared a lot of information with you. You do not have to do everything at once. I suggest that you start with one or two things and gradually add when you are ready. Let me repeat myself: This did not happen over night. It is a journey. Consistency is the most important thing you can do for yourself when making changes. You cannot do something for two to three days or even a week and expect to get the full results you are looking for and need. Stick with it, and I promise you will see the rewards of your labor.

August 2009 *It hasn't been that long since I was first diagnosed, and I know that I am moving in the right direction. Some friends visited me that haven't seen me in awhile, and they were surprised to see that I look better than when they last saw me, which was about five years ago. They kept saying, "This is not what I thought people looked like when they have been diagnosed with breast cancer." People are starting to have that aha moment, and are realizing that you don't have to brutally poison yourself to get better. Healing comes from God. Nutrition is just a bonus for you to live a long and healthy life. I don't know about you, but when I am ninety-nine, I want to be in my right mind and full of energy.*

I am still telling everyone that I am doing this the natural route.

Some thought it was great and others didn't. It's funny now, people don't even question what I am doing, because the truth speaks louder than the lies.

There have been some intense moments where I have been engulfed with fear. But when I wasn't fearful, I was almost euphoric. I know without a doubt I am going to walk this out with God by my side and tell everyone what He has done for me. I want others to know that my God heals and there are other options to treat cancer versus the conventional method.

Take time to discover the truth about your situation. Don't just believe everything you hear, even if it comes from a doctor. It's your job to be diligent in doing the research.

Discovery is the process of learning something, the fact or process of finding out about something for the first time.

Everybody wants to be a Healer

October 2009 *I stand firm in knowing that I have the right to choose what is best for my body. I do not have to forfeit my rights into the hands of a physician. This is a lot to process, plus I am still dealing with a lot of fear. Though I am fully aware of what the truth is, and I believe that God heals, I find myself grasping for straws and then I do something that is completely fear based. I think I am going to contact the healer my friend told me about during our trip to Mexico.*

I've searched all over for his phone number, but I can't find it.

Later *I was doing a little grocery shopping and as soon as I got back into my car, surprisingly there was the healer's number lying on the passenger seat. My initial reaction was that this is a sign from God! Even if it's not a sign, maybe He just wants me to experience this for myself in order to share what works and what doesn't. I am willing to do that.*

I made my appointment, and I set out on the adventure to

see what the fuss is all about. The healer's practice was located in a rented office space and those who come to see him are asked to make a donation for their healing appointments. I found him to be very humorous and extremely personable. Sitting on the table next to him was a picture of Jesus, and I thought to myself, "This is a good sign. Maybe he's actually a Christian."

As my session begins, he puts his hand over my breast (not touching it), and I could feel the heat from his hands. He then told me that he heals through angels and that we need to meet three times a week for the next six weeks in order for me to be fully healed. Logically, if he was an anointed healer, he would have just laid hands on me right then and there and I would have been healed instantly. That night I was really sick. When I told him what had happened, he said, "It's a good sign that my body was detoxing." Honestly, to this day, I really don't know what was wrong with me that particular evening.

November 2009 *I am sitting in the waiting room for my next appointment with the healer. There are a variety of people from all walks of life that are hoping this man will be able to heal them. He always says, "I will heal you," not that this is a gift from God, nor that God is working through me. It's was all about what he can do.*

I've started watching Christian men and women who are anointed healers on TV and online which helped me to better understand healing from a biblical standpoint. I have not yet seen an anointed man or woman of God heal in person. I do believe that Jesus heals and that He works through man to heal others, but man himself cannot heal alone. God has commissioned each of us to be His disciples and to go into the world declaring His glory. <u>Mark 16:15-18, (KJV)</u> – *"And he said unto them, Go ye into all the world, and preach the gospel to every creature. He that believeth and is baptized shall be saved; but he that believeth not shall be damned. And these signs shall follow them that believe… they shall lay hands on the sick and they shall recover."*

Later that month *I have been consistently going to this healer for a while, and I am still not healed. During one my visits, he made this crazy statement, "If you get pregnant, the cancer will go away." I thought this was absolutely absurd, because people get cancer even when they are pregnant. What in the world is he thinking?*

During the season of seeing him, he had moved into a new office space, and I finally realize what was going on. His new décor included Buda, the Indian god Lakshmi, pictures of yoga gurus, big crystals, plus a picture of Jesus. I started to understand that I was in the office of a metaphysical healer, who groups Jesus with all the other gods and healers. Even though I was more aware of his beliefs, I continued to see him.

During one visit, my curiosity began to stir and I started asking him questions about the angels he heals through and if he could describe them to me. He said sometimes he has to ask them to leave because they distract him and take his focus away. Things were just getting crazier and crazier to me. I was so amazed at how busy this man was, plus at how many people were willing to donate in order for him to build a healing center.

I had always avoided the group sessions, because I knew that some of the people would be too much for me. But one day, the only appointment I could get was a group session. You can't tell me God doesn't have a great sense of humor, because He was willing to let me go one step further before He stopped all this nonsense.

As I entered into the room everyone was gathered in a horseshoe shape sitting with the healer at the front of the group. All the people were lined up as he began his healing ritual and it was at this point, we all started getting hot. The healer could perform his ritual and talk at the same time. As things continued, I found myself caught up in the moment as I began to hear him make fun of the Pastor at the Baptist church, by saying that his nose and face were red and that he was going to buy his church building. Then others around me began to chime in and make remarks about this man of God. Some said he was an alcoholic. It made me so angry, that I looked at the healer and said, "Maybe he has rosacea." Then the lady close to me said, "Yeah, I'm a witch and I thought I was supposed to burn up when I walked into a church; Well I've never burned." Someone else made a comment about the Ft. Hood shootings and how the military was to blame for the gunman's actions. All of a sudden, all the witches started to come out and one asked, "What does give us this day our daily bread mean?"

It was at that moment that I became cold as ice. It was like I was covered in dry ice, I was freezing. I was completely separated from the group. I knew that God was saying "Venus, this is your last time, and I have separated you from them."

It was obvious that the healer knew something had happened because he kept looking at me, and I could sense he was very uncomfortable. I didn't even care. There was a boldness that had come over me, and I was not backing down. I believe in the supernatural—my angel and his demon were having it out. Guess who won!?!

As the healing session ended, I waited for the healer. I wanted to give him a piece of my mind. He tried hard to avoid me and told me he was in a hurry, but I was not letting him get away from me. I asked him why he would tell this friend of mine, who was very ill and has an illegitimate, handicapped child that if she got pregnant, she would get healed. I said to him, "Do you know what you could have done to her life, if she took your advice?" I went on to tell him, he had to take responsibility for his actions. He laughed and said, "I tell women in there seventies to get pregnant." I continued to tell him, he was not very responsible. He couldn't wait to get away from me, as he scurried off to his office with his false gods.

As soon as I got home, I called my friend, Kate and told her what had happened. She said, only the healer has the power to end a session and separate you from the group. I assured her that God decided to end the session on His time and that He is in charge of my life. When God says it's over, it's over.

I made sure she knew that I was never going back to see him again.

I have to admit, I'm a bit embarrassed that I told people about this guy because this is not of God. This healer was not the true HEALER, Jesus. I knew in my heart the truth, but fear was driving me to do other things I normally wouldn't do, and God allowed me to go there. He woke me up to see how the other side works and the lies that people fall for. I'm so thankful that He took me out of that whole ordeal just in the nick of time and said, "You've seen enough."

Still searching for answers, I was walking Iggy one day and I asked God for a sign to show me that I was on the right path. Psalm 23:2 dropped in my heart. As soon as I finished my walk, I immediately opened my Bible to read the scripture that God had dropped into my heart… Psalm 23:2 (NIV) – *"He makes me lie down in green pastures; he leads me beside quiet waters."* This was my sign, and I knew God was telling me and reminding me not to worry, that He was restoring me and that He would fulfill His word.

Psalm 23

"The Lord is my shepherd, I lack nothing. He makes me lie down in green pastures, he leads me beside quiet waters, he refreshes my soul. He guides me along the right paths for his name's sake. Even though I walk through the darkest valley, I will fear no evil for you are with me; your rod and your staff, they comfort me. You prepare a table before me in the presence of my enemies. You anoint my head with oil; my cup overflows. Surely goodness and

love will follow me all the days of my life, and I will dwell in the house of the Lord forever."

If you have been diagnosed with cancer and fear is trying to consume you, I want you to know that God restores, He refreshes, and He heals. Don't allow fear to take flight in your heart and mind, instead allow Him to lead you beside still waters, and He will quiet your heart.

There is only one God, and I can testify to His faithfulness. He does indeed heal!

Saint Janelle and the TaTa Sisterhood 2010

"I haven't seen you in a while, yet I often imagine all your expressions. I haven't spoken to you recently, but many times I hear your thoughts. Good friends must not always be together. It is the feeling of oneness, when distant that proves a lasting."

- Unknown

July 2010 *I love Austin!*

I know I keep saying it over and over again, but I really do love this place. When something like cancer strikes, you find out quickly who your real friends are. I feel so blessed to have such incredible friends, both locally and across the United States, who have been by my side each step of the way. There have been days when someone would just call to say hello or to offer a word of encouragement that would brighten my day. Others took time out of their busy schedules to drop by for a visit, to show their care and concern. To all my friends, who stood in the *gap for me, I love you and I want you to know how much your friendship has meant to me. Proverbs 18:24 (MSG) – "Friends come and friends go, but a true friend sticks by you like family." You see, I found cancer to be a very lonely disease, especially in the beginning when I was trying to figure things out. At least it was for me.*

But let's get back to the Ta Ta Sisterhood. My friend Janelle, who looks like a tall sexy Shirley Temple is what I call a super friend. She is someone who is always there for you and has a very special way of gathering people together, that's why I have given her the name, Saint Janelle.

After a year of exploring all the good and bad treatments available for breast cancer and being a human guinea pig, money was running out and debt was piling up. Saint Janelle and a group of women called the Femtastics—a group I joined to meet new people—develop new relationships and network. Even though the group broke apart after a year, several of us remained friends. These women decided to rally together and host a fundraising event just for me. Thus was the introduction of the Ta Ta Sisterhood.

I had such mixed emotions about allowing the Ta Ta Sisterhood to do this for me. I knew I needed financial help, and I also wanted to get the message out to those who have been diagnosed with breast cancer; there are other options available to them. I was worried and a bit embarrassed about what other people would think and concerned if anyone would actually show up for the event.

I have always been the one to give to others, so learning to receive has been a hard lesson for me. I am teaching myself that there are seasons in life where we need to enjoy both giving and receiving. If someone offers to give you something, don't steal the blessing away from them by not graciously accepting their gift with a heart of gratitude.

With great anticipation, the day of the Ta Ta Sisterhood fundraiser finally arrived. I was so excited I could hardly contain myself. My prayer was to have grace to handle myself well and share the message God had put on my heart. This was one of the best days of my life and it was time to put my receiver on! I selected a really cute dress and smashing pair of sandals for the event. Just a quick side note – rayon and polyester blend (no matter how cute) are not a good idea in the Texas heat. The material doesn't breathe and all you do is sweat, not perspire, and sweat!

I was completely overwhelmed with emotions as I arrived at the event. The Ta Ta Sisterhood knows how to throw one heck of a party and this was the first fundraising event they had ever done. Three snaps up in a circle for The Ta Ta Sisterhood! They thought of everything from food, live music, silent and live auctions, even entertainment for the kids. I couldn't believe how many people showed up, even ones that didn't know me. Some of my wonderful friends from out of town, Victor, Shelly and Ellen made the trip to be there and celebrate with me. My sweet neighbor Kambi came with her mother and aunt. I love her family so much! Her mom, Cindy was there for me a year ago when I was in a car accident, right before I was leaving for Mexico. She is so kind and comforting. She just hugged me and let me weep. Thank-you Cindy! People I hadn't seen in years came out to support me. But little did I know during all of this, that someone was walking away upset with me.

Joel McColl, Lorrie Sanger, and the Sarah Pierce Band kept the place jamming with some great music all through out the evening. As I think back to this day, I still get overwhelmed with emotion. This event had it all from food, friends, and entertainment, not to mention what a huge financial blessing it was to me. I have never felt so loved and encouraged before.

As I was chatting with everyone and taking pictures, I realized that some actually thought I had gone the conventional route. I'm sure they wondered why I had hair and looked so healthy.

By now, I'm chomping at the bit and I can't wait to give my speech. I am scheduled to give a speech, Is It the Fear or the Disease, in Florida within a couple of weeks. This would be the very first time for me to speak in front of a group and share what was on my heart, so the next 15 minutes is the start of something great.

Later *It felt so good! This is right where I want to be, in front of people, telling my truth, sharing God's truth and giving them hope while letting them see that you can heal without surgery, poisoning, or burning their bodies. If just one person walked away with the truth, it was a success.*

After the fundraiser concluded that night, I went home and stayed up for hours talking to my dear friend Victor. Everything was still so surreal. Never had anyone done something so significant for me. When I finally went to bed, all I could think about was the speech I was going to give at the T-Tapp retreat, in Florida. I knew this was my calling, to share the truth with others. Would I choke or not be able to speak in front of others, would they cry or laugh, and could I get the message across to them about the seriousness of taking care of their health? I sure hoped so. I knew without a doubt that God had called me to share the truth with others.

As far as the person who got upset with me at my fundraiser, are you for real!?! Someone is always trying to steal your thunder. The next day I got an email from this friend who thought I didn't want her to be at the fundraiser. I just don't understand how stuff like this happens in the midst of a special moment. My email response was simple and straight to the point, "Couldn't you tell how excited I was to see you?" I hadn't seen her in years. I even offered to have lunch, so we could have some one-on-one time, but she never responded. I was truly sorry she left feeling hurt like she did. But you know there is always someone that has themselves on their mind 24/7 and this wasn't going to steal my joy. I wanted to share the moments of the fundraiser with everyone who came out to show their support.

Friends, there are nothing like them!

"Friends are like bras; close to your heart and there for support." - Unknown

To the Ta Ta Sisterhood, I love you!

"A true friend knows the song in my heart and sings it to me when my memory fails."

- Donne Roberts

Defeating Your Goliaths

June, 2010. *Today is the day that I begin this chapter about my battle with my own personal Goliath. I've gone back and forth about sharing this very personal, private information in this book but I honestly believe that in order to be healed we have to be healed emotionally as well as physically so with tears streaming down my face I'm going ahead with writing about it.*

Emotional enemies are deep wounds of the heart and soul where we have been traumatized by someone or something along life's journey. Some people call facing these emotional enemies *dealing with your demons* but I prefer to call it *Facing Your Goliaths* because of one of my all-time favorite Bible stories.

I Samuel 17 tells how David, as a young man, defeated Goliath, a 10 feet tall giant, using only three small stones and a slingshot. Not only did David not turn tail and run away, he bravely ran toward something much larger than himself and defeated the giant that stood there.

We all have giants to face in our lives. These *Goliaths* come in various shapes and sizes and include things like divorce, loss of a loved one, sexual, emotional and physical abuse or even an array of other failures and disappointments. It is so much easier to run from the giants than to face them but avoidance only brings a false sense of peace and harmony. We think that *ignorance is bliss* but in reality not dealing with these *Goliaths* only ends up making both our emotional and physical self completely toxic. Thoughts generate 98% of disease and 98% of all disease is avoidable; therefore, it is vital that you deal with what is eating at you on the inside.

When you are young and adored by everyone, it is easy to trust in people. After all isn't that the great thing about being a child, your innocence. Unfortunately, there are people who have something dark inside them - their own Goliath if you will. I believe that these kinds of people need to control their environment at all times even at the expense of a child.

When I was in seventh grade I was left alone with someone - I was around 12 or 13 at the time - and still vividly remember every detail of what happened - even down to what I was wearing that day. All I need to say bad things were done to me that day. I will spare you the details because even after all this time, they are enough to make me ill. As a young, frightened girl, I couldn't understand what had just happened to me and I honestly didn't know what to do.

I did tell another adult that I trusted what had happened and I believe that this is what saved me from more harm from this person in the ensuing years even though the other adult never uttered a word in my defense. This other person, that I trusted enough to tell of this horrific incident, did nothing but stand there in silence.

I still cannot comprehend why I was never comforted about what happened and was left alone to deal with all the emotions that I was feeling. This lack of action left me even more confused and hurt than ever because I now had to deal with the worst kind of betrayal from two adults I trusted - one who took horrible advantage of me and one who stood by and did nothing. I was sure of one thing, and that was that I would *never* allow anyone to do that to me again. I know that a lot of young people who are victims of bad things are convinced that they did something wrong or something to deserve it but I never thought it was my fault and knew absolutely that what had happened to me was wrong.

As I got older this persons anger escalated toward me whenever we were together. I think that they believed that they were under the microscope and that their behavior was being watched by others even though no one had done anything to stop or report them. Looking back on these things it's hard not to feel a deep sense of sadness and betrayal from the Dr. Jekyll/Mr. Hyde personality this person had exhibited throughout my life. I never knew if they were going to be fun, kind, encouraging or the exact opposite whenever I ran into them.

Although I had times of normalcy and even happy memories

in my life after that, I was never comfortable around this person and continually walked on egg shells trying to gauge their emotional status. I truly believe this persons guilt was causing a Goliath to start rising.

I honestly believe that this event caused me to search for love in all the wrong places and ways. At the time I didn't realize that I was in search of something but looking back I am keenly aware of my actions. By the time I was fifteen I was partying hard. I finished High School while shoving most of these emotions deep down, playing volleyball, basketball and dreaming of my future.

I moved across country to California and became busy establishing myself as an Esthetician. I launched several new businesses, built friendships, fell in love and got married. After five years, my marriage came to a screeching halt and we divorced and went our separate ways.

During all of this time it was nice to be on the opposite coast away from the scarred childhood memories that now lived only deep within my heart. I was in control of when I wanted to go and see everyone and could stay as long or as short of a time as I wanted to.

By the time I had moved on with my life, I heard this person had become much more openly rude to other people around him. Prior to this point, I heard he was able to control his behavior in front of others. He was so good at hiding it that no one would believe me when I told them he was nuts but it was obvious to me that one day, this giant secret was going to explode.

On rare occasions people from my past would visit me in California and one time it was the woman who had walked away and failed to protect me when I asked for help. I was giving her a facial and talking about some of the horrible things that had happened to me that had been swept under the rug. Her response was "Oh Venus, just let it go. You will be surprised at what you can let go." I then asked her what I wanted to ask for years. "Why didn't anyone ever help me? Her answer was "I told him if he ever hurt you again, I would call the police". That was nice to know but certainly would have been nicer if I had been told that back when it had happened. It would have been even nicer to know that someone validated my feelings and agreed that what had happened was wrong.

If I had only been given the protection that I needed and deserved, things would have been so different but the person that I trusted to tell what was going on had a philosophy that ignoring something meant that it didn't happen. Maybe she honestly didn't know how to protect me and sometimes I wonder if she was left to fend for herself as a child as well.

My *Goliath* has gotten even crazier and more controlling over the years and now has no problem ranting and raving in front of other people. Even when other people comment on the verbal abuse it still continued. During a visit I saw these examples first hand and it took me a solid month to get over this trip. I became depressed and started struggling with all those horrid, haunting memories of childhood all over again.

During another trip a few years later, I saw this person and was reminded again that some people do everything that they can to control their environment and the people in their lives but now the giant was coming out of the closet and this person was no longer able to control their behavior in front of anyone. He had become quite offensive and would very often say inappropriate things to people - especially women - and even throw frequent tantrums in public. As usual there were some who continued to smile and behave as if nothing were wrong thinking that if they were nice enough, others would overlook the horrid behavior of this person.

I finally decided that I couldn't be around this person anymore. Just dealing with this personality on infrequent phone calls had the ability to throw me into a full blown anxiety attack. Although this person continued to try to get back into contact with me in order to control me again, I didn't waiver on my decision and for the first time in my life I started to feel in control.

Fast forward a few years to April, 2009 when I was diagnosed with breast cancer. My head was spinning and all I could think about is how much I needed support.

Even though I let everyone in my life know that I was going to go an alternative route for my healing and that I would not be having surgery or chemo, some people never believed me with one or the other calling to talk me out of my decision and to go a more traditional route for dealing with cancer. It had been a good five years since I had seen or spoken to the person who had taken advantage of me as a girl and I wasn't ready yet to deal with all of that because I was trying to keep my stress levels as low as possible in order to heal.

It was during this journey of healing that I realized I did, in fact, have to face my Goliath and defeat him - all by myself. It was time to stop running. I had to figure out how to forgive this person for what had been done to me. You see, the pain that I had experienced from that day caused me to be physically sick and I had never addressed it - only allowed it to eat away at me from the inside for years. I knew this wasn't going to be easy but I wanted to be healthy again. No more running away.

Forgiveness doesn't just happen though, no matter how bad you want it to. It is a process - sometimes a very long one - and I worked hard at learning how to forgive. Slowly, as time went on, my heart was softening and I realized that I was beginning to forgive him. The uncomfortable feelings were slowly being replaced with compassion toward this person.

You may not understand why I forgave him and you may not believe that you can forgive the past hurts in your own life but the truth is that the only person that you hurt when you don't forgive someone is yourself. The person who has hurt you has moved on from the point of pain while you continue to stand in the midst of the hurt many years later. Forgiving someone else for their wrongs against you should be done for your own well being. It brings about healing and restoration both physically and mentally. Remember that God has forgiven you for much and in the same manner we are expected to forgive others no matter how great the hurt. It doesn't mean that we say that the previous behavior is okay, it just means that we forgive and we move on in a healthy state of mind.

In October of 2010 I was invited to a fitness retreat hosted by muscle activation specialist Teresa Tapp to speak on a topic that is near and dear to my heart...."Is it the Fear of the Disease?" This was the time and opportunity that I needed - not only to speak and share with others the wonderful things God has shown me on my journey - but also I needed to face my Goliath who was residing nearby. I knew that if I wanted to be completely healed I had to face my giant.

I had absolutely no fear or anxiety in going to visit this time around. Some of my acquaintances were very uptight about it all. Some of the others were living in the land of denial - the place where everything is fine and nothing could ever go wrong. You know, just keep smiling and everything will be OK.

As for me? I was glad to see everyone and for some reason I laughed the whole time I as there. Psalm 16:9 - "Therefore my heart is glad and my glory (my inner self) rejoices; my body too shall rest and confidently dwell in safety." For the first time in my life, this person's behavior didn't bother me at all. God had enabled me to change my thoughts and the way that I felt toward him. He had miraculously made it possible for me to truly forgive him so that I could find peace within myself and not be affected by his behavior anymore.

When we were leaving a friend told me that I had handled the situation so much better than they had and I was able to share with her that this was all God's doing and how He had changed me so that I could come out on the other side of the fire strong and whole. Philippians 4:13 - "I can do all things through Christ who strengthens me."

Since the breast cancer diagnosis I have done several different detox programs in order to rid my body of toxins so by now my body was pretty clean. For some reason I decided to do another six-week detox for my colon, kidneys, liver, gallbladder and my blood but during this particular detox I found myself much more easily agitated and angry. I am usually full of life and a very happy-go-lucky person and anger is not the norm for me. Little did I know that God was using this particular detox to bring about a complete spiritual detox as well.

A few weeks later the woman I had asked for help called, and I told her that I still didn't understand why she hadn't stood up for me when I was a child when I had told her I needed help. She was crying just asking for forgiveness over and over stating that she just didn't have enough self esteem to stand up for me.

At that moment I had an epiphany. I realized for the first time that I had even more anger built up against her than the person who had done such horrible things to me. I expressed to her how angry I was that she hadn't stood up for me all those years ago. I told her that children *must* be put first and taken care of no matter what.

The next day I was trying to use my copier and it didn't do what I wanted it to do. All of a sudden something snapped in me and all the years of bottled up anger at this person who left me to fend for myself took over as I slammed the copier on the floor, jumped up and down on it, beat it and threw it against the wall. I tore that copier to pieces so bad that my poor dog ran and hid because he had never seen me behave like this. I was running outside with pieces of the copier and throwing them on the front lawn. I didn't even know that I was strong enough to do the damage that I did but when it was all said and done, I felt like the weight of the world had been lifted off my shoulders. My friends still joke about the copier saying that it was like a scene from the TV sitcom *The Office*. I always seem to do these strange, crazy things in moments of stress in my life.

The next day my dog walker was talking about how smashed up the copier on the front lawn was and that it was so mangled that it looked like someone had thrown it from the top floor of the apartment unit. He went on to say that the weird thing about it was that my dog had insisted on walking over to it and peeing on it. I laughed so hard that I almost cried while I told him that it was my copier and my dog was apparently saying, "piss on you copier for making my mom so mad."

So when everything was said and done I realized, after all

these years, that my actual Goliath was not who I originally thought but rather the person I had asked for help because she never stood up for or protected me. My anger towards her was more intense because I knew that the person who had hurt me was probably mentally ill. God had helped me find a way to forgive him and now I needed His help again in finding a way to forgive her as well. I started this process with forgiveness affirmations every day saying "I forgive you, I love you and I bless you." This may sound corny to you but this is what I really did and you know what? After saying something repeatedly it actually becomes the truth and I was able to forgive her.

In order to defeat your own *Goliaths*, you must figure out what the issues of *your* heart are and what's really eating at you on the inside. In order to heal emotionally and physically you need to address these wounds that you have buried away deep within yourself.

When I interview women who have come to me for help in healing their breast cancer the first question I ask them is what they think the root cause of their diagnosis is. The number one response I get is stress.

The most interesting discovery that I find when I uncover the deep issues of the heart with these women is that most of them have experienced a bad relationship or there was someone who had hurt them deeply that they had never been able to forgive. Any painful experience can create a lack of trust and according to Dr. Alex Loyd, author of the bestselling book *The Healing Code*, breast cancer is a trust and patience issue. Trust is the absolute biggest issue that has to be dealt with when it comes to breast cancer.

As for me, I believe that breast cancer is also a matter of the heart. Think about it. The breast is where your heart lies, you feed your children from your breasts and when your children hurt themselves they lay their head against your chest and you stroke their back and tell them that everything is going to be okay. Everything about the breast area of your body has to do with nurturing. A broken heart can definitely lead to physical and emotional disease.

You will never heal unless you defeat your own Goliath. Remember that it is faster and easier to go through the mountain than the long way around it. To heal physically you must get to the emotional root of the problem.

Dr. Caroline Leaf, author of the *Switch On Your Brain 5 Step Learning Process* program says, "Every gene lies dormant until a thought activates it." My breast didn't cause the cancer to come so cutting them off just wasn't logical to me. I had to determine what thoughts I had that cancer would come to my breast and I found that being unable or unwilling to forgive certain people was the root of my own problem.

Every trauma we have in our life - physical or emotional - will sit in our cells and our cells have memory. You *have* to deal with the cell memory. For example, I didn't even realize that my anger was directed at a completely different person than I originally thought. She was a person that always seemed like a victim herself and this brought out my own protective instincts making me feel sorry for her and that I had to protect her instead of realizing that, as an adult, it was *her* job to protect me - the child.

Once I finally figured out what was eating on me from the inside and addressed it, I was able to begin building healthy relationships accepting them for what they are. It is so refreshing to be able to have relationships with everyone without expectations from them. God has granted me compassion and proven to me that forgiveness must be given to those that wrong us in order to heal yourself and promote your own wellbeing.

Just remember that you can't cut, poison or burn yourself to solve the root of your problem. That only gets rid of the physical manifestation of the problem not the problem itself. A lot of people treat the symptoms which is the cancer, by going either the natural or conventional route, but they fail to address the root of the problem and without that, the symptom itself will resurface again and again.

The good news is that there are many tools available to assist you when dealing with your own emotional and physical *Goliaths*. I recommend prayer, devotional time, finding a local church or spiritual group that can help support you emotionally and seeing a good counselor that can properly direct you. I also recommend reading *The Healing Code*. If done consistently and properly you will find great peace in utilizing these codes.

Proverbs 3:5-6 - "Trust in the Lord with all your heart, and do not lean on your own understanding; in all your ways acknowledge Him and He will make your paths straight." Ask God to give you the wisdom and ability to work through your problems. Learn to trust again starting with God because He is the one who will never fail you.

The truth will set you free. God's word says that in Him and knowing Him is freedom and it was for freedom of our souls that Jesus died. The whole purpose of defeating your *Goliath* is so that God's healing balm will cure the sickness of the soul.

I Samuel 17:45 - "Then said David to Goliath, You come to me with a sword, a spear and a javelin but I come to you in the name of the Lord." Just like David, with God on your side, you *can* defeat your own *Goliath*.

It is very important to me to close out this chapter with a warning to all adults about the importance of protecting children from harm. It is the adults absolute responsibility to address any concerns or situations any child brings to their attention. Don't ignore or minimize the problem and think it will go away. You must investigate any incidents thoroughly and take them seriously. God gave us stewardship over children to raise them in a healthy and secure environment.

I can now close this chapter of my life no longer running away from the giants in my life for my *Goliath* has been defeated.

A letter is an important way to say what you want to say

whether you end up giving it to the person or burning it ceremonially. Either way you are getting rid of the toxic effect on your body by saying it out loud. Here is a letter that I sent. Although I kept mine short and sweet, you can use it as a template - expanding and changing as needed - for your own letter.

Dear ---------,

I send you this letter to remind you and make sure that you know that I have forgiven you for everything you have done in the past. Though there were difficult times that we went through, I do recognize and see the good parts of you too. Now it's time for you to ask God for forgiveness and forgive yourself.

Love,

Venus

"You God, are a healing balm and your grace is a medicine that we can apply to our hearts that brings forth spiritual and emotional healing."

- Lisa Smith

Is It the Fear or the Disease?

Cancer. Just saying this word can create fear in a person's heart. People immediately think worst-case scenario when this word is spoken over them.

When a victim of cancer has the difficult task of informing friends and family of their diagnosis, the automatic reaction they receive is one of compassion and sorrow. Staring face to face with those they love, fear exudes immediately from their eyes. Yes, that four letter word, FEAR, quickly overtakes them. You wonder, are they praying at that moment not to become a victim themselves, or are they hoping one of these so called Special Interest groups will finally develop a cure instead of handing over years of empty promises once again?

The question stirs so deeply within me when I see so many people participating in these pink events. How many more walks do they think they have to attend and how many more pink ribbon products do they think they have to purchase before there's a cure? I believe that women in the pink club secretly think if they exhaust all efforts in working hard to raise money for the cure, they will earn extra karma points and if by chance they are diagnosed there will soon be a cure. All this pink, yet NO CURE! Please don't misunderstand me, I honestly get why so much energy and effort is put toward this cause, it's because women are extremely compassionate and sympathetic and they truly want to help.

I certainly hope after reading my book, someone will be inspired to start working passionately to promote the nonprofits organizations that generously give to those who wish to choose the natural route, but do not have the financial means to do so. You may not be aware that insurance companies do not cover alternative treatments; they only pay for conventional treatments. I feel that a lot of people choose the conventional method not only because of fear, but also due to that fact that their insurance will partially pay for the treatment.

I am working diligently to establish a nonprofit organization that will assist those who have been diagnosed with cancer, and to help others who want to make preventive lifestyle changes in regards to their health. I have learned so much on this journey and I refuse to sit back timidly and watch others be overtaken by fear. I want to share the wealth of knowledge I have gained because people deserve to know the truth – THERE ARE OTHER OPTIONS available.

Don't let fear drive your decisions! Did you know, when a person is delivered a diagnosis, or told there is a chance they may have cancer, their cortisol levels rise so high it can put the body into death mode. 2 Timothy 1:7 – *"For God has not given us a spirit of fear but of power and of love and of a sound mind."*

I have asked myself this question, why do we look at cancer the way we do? Think about for a moment. What we know about cancer has been carefully put together by the pharmaceutical industry and media propaganda, which is intended to keep us in the dark about the amazing superiority of Mother Nature to heal cancer.

What is Cancer? Well to begin with, it's a multibillion-dollar business! I'm here to tell you cancer is alive and well on planet earth. Did you know a woman with breast cancer is worth 800,000 to 1 million dollars to the medical system? Even with the billions of dollar poured into research a year, western medicine has only improved cancer survival rates by only 2.3 to 5% in the last 55 years. These startling statistics should stir you to be proactive in your health, creating a desire within you to develop good habits that can prevent cancer.

How about looking at it from this perspective, if 2,600 woman get breast cancer and they chose the medical route of chemo, surgery and possibly radiation, five years later only 36 will be alive. Let me leave this nugget for your to ponder upon as well, there is no cure for chemo! So, the choice is yours today, do you want sit idle by waiting for a cure?

I believe that prevention is the only sensible thing for a person to do. There are many doctors who offer alternative cancer treatments. These physicians are forced to treat their patients outside of the United States, because the alternative treatment is considered illegal here in the U.S. What a crying shame that in the land of the free we are not allowed to choose our own method of medical treatment.

What if we looked at cancer in a different light? If it is a biological process that requires certain conditions for the process to operate and tumors are the symptoms and products of this process - cancer is not the tumor, but the process that is producing the tumor. By the time the tumor is diagnosed you have had cancer for years, maybe decades. The important thing to do is to shut down the process. People are fooled into thinking if they cut, burn or poison the body, the process will be shut down. This is not the case. Conventional treatment only takes care of the symptoms, not the cause, leaving a vast opportunity for the cancer to return even stronger the second time around.

Statistically a true cure rate of 90% is achieved by cancer patients who avoid orthodox medicine and go the alternative route. If those who chose the natural route stay consistent with their preventive health measures and continue to do their homework along the way they will reap the healthy benefits from their due diligence. I will take those odds any day over 2.3 to 5% survival rates for the conventional method. Chemo not only severely damages the body, but those who fall prey to it will more than likely see the cancer return down the road and be stronger and more violent than before. I talk to people all the time that have experienced this to be true. I just met a woman recently, who had been diagnosed with stage one breast cancer and she chose the conventional route. After going through surgery and chemo with the first diagnosis, she was then given a clean bill of health for a short period of time. Upon returning to the doctor for a checkup, she was informed that the cancer had returned with a vengeance and had spread to her liver, into her lymphatic system and is now stage four cancer. Guess what she decided to do? She went back for more! More burning, more poison, more hopeless promises from the medical society. Maybe this time it will cure her. My hope and prayer is that these statistics will alarm you more than the fear you become consumed with when you are diagnosed. Allow the fear to drive you down a healthy path – turn your fear into a walk of faith.

Why are people so convinced that conventional treatments are the only way to go? Here are some of reasons I think people choose the way they do:

- Medical Professionals are addicted to using drugs to cure a problem (in this case cancer) instead of finding ways of prevention. Cancer patients themselves contribute to the problem. They feel that if there was a cure for cancer their doctor would know about it, so they assume a cure doesn't exist and they fail to research all the options available to them. The doctor becomes their god.

- Medical professionals are addicted to the thought that they are the only qualified ones with the answers. This is not the case, because I have met some amazing doctors who offer alternative treatments and made significant changes to the way they treat their patients. They have discovered the truth when it comes to conventional vs. natural methods of treatment.

- Once again it comes back to money! The pharmaceutical companies want patients (consumers) to try and cure themselves through medication, not prevention and holistic treatments because every person who gets cancer increase's the shareholders value.

Does this sound harsh? I hope so! Maybe someone reading this will open their eyes, minds and hearts, and get proactive about their own personal health prevention.

If disease is a biological process, it can be turned on and it can be turned off. We should be looking at this from a different angle. From my own personal experience and all of the research I have done, I believe that disease or health issues are just malfunctioning oxygen depleted cells.

There are many pathways to becoming imbalanced. Dr Andreas Moritz believes that cancer is a survival mechanism of the body. Its saying stop with all the bad habits, I'm on toxic overload, it's time to turn the switch "off". But most people want the magic little pill, instead of changing their lifestyles. That always amazes me, because I truly want to live my life and live it to the fullest. If only everyone would do their homework, how eye opening it would be.

Ann Wigmore and many others in the health field (not the death field) profession have said deficiency and toxemia are the causes of all disease. Cleanse the body and the mind, so the body will heal itself. We must never forget the past, before the 1940's we were a healthier people. Our food was real and we didn't consume the large amounts of sugar and junk food as we do today. There weren't pesticides, dyes, chemicals, drug therapies and definitely no GMO foods like we have today. People were much more connected; they valued God, country and family to a higher degree. Today, we live such fast paced lives, always on the go, eating on the go, always connected to some kind of technical device and we are no longer paying attention to what's most important. No wonder cancer and disease is at an epidemic proportion!

I want to remind you of the most important thing of all, God almighty created these bodies and He does all things perfectly. We are meant to function in wholeness and perfect health just the way we were created. I believe one day in the future people will look back on how cancer was treated and think "how barbaric" just the way we look at bloodletting.

I am going to say it again Prevention is the key! Stand up for your rights to have organic real food not the genetically modified foods which are being sold inexpensively so everyone can afford it in our supermarkets. I beg of you to say No to this monstrosity of frankenfoods.

Let me close with this thought for you to really ponder ... *"Is it the fear or the disease"*? What's driving you to make the decisions you are making concerning your health? The fear of a health crisis should drive you to making healthy lifestyle changes instead of choosing a treatment that continues to break your body down.

Remember to pause first, get away if you can, and remove the fear and those around you who are fearful. Pray and seek God for wisdom concerning your health, then make the right decision concerning your well being.

Ecclesiastes 7:11-13 (AMPL) – "For wisdom is a defense even as money is a defense, but the excellency of knowledge is that wisdom shields and preserves the life of him who has it."

Let knowledge and wisdom be the key to your health success. Replace fear with blind faith, I am living proof that it will lead you to a path of healing and wholeness.

Psalm 37:4 Delight yourself in the Lord and he will give you the desires of your heart.

Remarkable Paths

Remarkable: to be worthy of notice or commenting on. The remarkable journey I have been on for the last couple of years is full of incredible, sometime intense moments, yet it is filled with God's love and direction, as well as new relationships that have enhanced each day of my life. I wish I could share every experience with you. Here are some of the highlights I think you will enjoy reading about.

Remarkable relationships. The relationships I made in the past couple of years are connections that put me in touch with critical people who had valuable knowledge and expertise that I could apply to my health. Some of those relationships were also cultivated into friends that I will cherish for a lifetime.

Dr. Hines, an intelligent, caring physician that I am so grateful to have met, imparted a wealth of information to me pertaining to my health. I always enjoyed contacting his office, and talking to his wife. During one of our conversations, she provided me with a contact she thought would be beneficial to me, Michelle Hart who owns a Thermography company called DITI Imaging (www.ditiimaging.com). Networking and connections indeed prove to be powerful tools. One call led to another, then to another... What an array of wonderful people!

I contacted Michelle and gathered details from her regarding DITI Imaging Company and shared my story with her. During our conversation, she told me about a dear friend of hers, Chris Templeton, who once was an actress on the well known soap, *The Young and the Restless*. From a young age, Chris suffered from polio, yet overcame all obstacles and was one of the first successful handicapped actresses. At this season of her life, Chris had been battling cancer for close to ten years. She was so warm and caring which made it easy for our friendship to blossom so quickly. During one of our chats, she shared her own personal health struggles as well as the passion she had to help others in need. Her compassion for those fighting cancer inspired her to start a foundation called, RAWtatoilli, which delivered raw food to cancer patients. Remarkable!

One day I decided that I wanted to meet this lovely lady in person, so I took a trip to down to San Antonio, which is a hop, skip and jump from Austin. While I was there, she shared with me her plans to travel over all of U.S. in search of treatments that would cure her. We were always each other cheerleaders, rooting for each other to be healed and healthy once again.

The pressure and stress seemed too much for her most of the time as she continued her search for treatments that might improve her health. In an effort to do something special for Chris, I decided to donate ten percent of the proceeds from the fundraiser my friends threw for me. I knew this would allow her to receive some special IV treatments that she really needed. Unfortunately Chris' health took a downhill spiral and she's now cheering me and her loved ones on as she smiles down from Heaven pain free, healed and whole.

Connection means to link an association between people, things or events. One day at the office, I was reviewing a consultation sheet from one of my clients. She indicated that she regularly does a T-Tapp workout. Curiously, I asked what that is. She explains that T-Tapp is a nuerokentic compound muscle workout mainly targeting the lymphatic system. This triggered an interest within me, because of the line of work I am in as an Esthetician. Later when I had the chance, I did some additional research on Teresa Tapp's website to learn more about this routine and her products. Another remarkable connection made! The information I found was fascinating and enlightening. I ordered several of her beginner videos and I still today enjoy doing the T-Tapp workout. I highly recommend that you take some time to familiarize yourself with her and the amazing tools and work shops she offers. (www.t-tapp.com).

Teresa Tapp, beautiful, inspiring, intelligent, full of life and energy has certainly blessed me beyond words. One day I received an email from Teresa inviting me to share my speech

"Is it the Fear or the Disease" at one of her beauty boot camps. I gladly accepted the invitation. I can't express how excited I was about this golden opportunity. I had no earthly idea if I would be a great public speaker or not, the only thing I knew for sure is that God had given me this chance to share a message with others that could change their lives. He chose me for this particular time! God chose me – what a privilege and honor that He trusts me that much.

October 2010 *The time finally arrived for me to hop on a plane and head to Florida to speak at the beauty boot camp. Not only am I thrilled about my speaking engagement, but my sister and her best friend are joining me at the event. What an adrenaline rush—I love every single minute of it! It's the first time giving my speech to a crowd.*

The feedback I received was so amazing and encouraged me so much! A brand new beginning and I knew that this was exactly what I wanted to do. I want to inspire others to take care of themselves, be proactive with their health, and prevent disease by sharing my story and the wealth of information I have obtained along the way. Remarkable future!

After the retreat concluded, we are all gathered in the bar area downstairs at the hotel. Let me set the stage for you before I go any further. A few months prior to this speaking engagement, I was watching Sid Roth, who host a show called It's Supernatural. (www.sidroth.org). on this particular show his guest was a Pastor by the name of Billy Burke. Pastor Billy shared how he was healed of cancer by Kathryn Kuhlman.

As a young man, he had been diagnosed with brain cancer and was given only three weeks to live. His grandmother, who knew the Great Physician (God), could do anything, decided to take him to a service where Kathryn Kuhlman was ministering. That evening, Kathryn laid hands on him and he was immediately healed. That miraculous event changed his life forever. From that time on Pastor Billy continued to study under Kathryn leadership until she passed away. He now travels worldwide preaching about God's grace and His healing power.

The Remarkable Healer! If you are not familiar with the Bible, I hope that you will take some time to research the information I am sharing with you. Matthew 4:23 - *"Jesus went throughout Galilee, teaching in their synagogues, preaching the good news of the kingdom, and healing every disease and sickness among the people."* You may ask does Jesus still heal today. The answer to your question is yes He does. Hebrews 13:8: *"Jesus Christ is the same yesterday and today and forever."* Healing applies to us today.

I was completely mesmerized by this show and how God healed him. I immediately went online to gather more details about his ministry. To my surprise his ministry was located in Tampa, Florida which is twenty minutes outside of where I would be speaking. I wondered if I would have the opportunity to actual meet him while I was in Florida.

I love how God directs our footsteps. There we were gathering in the bar area of the hotel, the featured speakers and those who put the amazing boot camp together. As I enter into the bar, I literally sat down next to a lady named, Shelly Ballestero, (www.beautybygodbook.com) who also spoke at the event. She immediately said to me, "you're the real thing." Would you by chance be interested in meeting Pastor Billy Burke? I had said nothing to her about Billy Burke, nor did I even know that she knew him. I asked her, "How do you know Billy Burke"? She told me that her husband was the head worship leader for his ministry. Coincidence? Not at all! Remarkable God. I told her that I just watched him on a segment of the Sid Roth show. We quickly made plans to meet Saturday night and attend one of his services. I was so excited that I told an older couple from Minnesota I had met about it. They too were big fans of his and asked if they could join us.

October 2010 *Saturday night is finally here. As we were driving to the church that evening, I had these preconceived ideas, thinking he must Pastor a huge church since he travels constantly speaking to thousands. But in actuality he ministers to a local church of approximately 100 people that have service in a meeting room at a Marriott. It was not what I had expected, but miracles can happen anywhere. Jesus was always en route somewhere when he encountered someone in need of a healing touch.*

As we entered into the room, Shelly took us directly to the front row, where her husband Angelo had reserved seating for us. As the service begin, it was a bit different and on a smaller scale than what I was used to. There were no Teleprompters, the band was smaller and they sang a lot of the older hymns of which I did not know. The older couple I was sitting with knew all the songs and words. I didn't care, every time I heard the word Jesus, I would raise my hand and say Jesus. It didn't stop me from thoroughly enjoying myself.

We had the best seats in house. Pastor Billy was right in my face. He's such a dynamic preacher! As he concluded his message, he looked over at the older couple I was sitting with and asked them to stand up. As they went forward, he prayed for Sam first, barely touching his forehead, the man hits the floor, slain in the spirit. Pastor Billy then prays for Abigail and the same thing happens to her. The presence of God was so strong that night! As I am standing there in my dress, I turn to the man behind me that I call a "catcher" and said, "Whatever happens, don't let my dress fly up."

Suddenly, I hear Shelly's husband, Angelo tell me to get over here and have him pray for me. The older couple on the floor is now coming back to their senses and return to their seats. Pastor Billy continues to ignore me while he is praying for others. He finally walks over to me and say's "what do you need God to do in your life?" I tell him about the large tumor in my breast. He asked me what stage of breast cancer and I told him it didn't matter, I just want it gone! It was time for this to be over! He begins to pray over me and lightly touches my forehead and down I go to the floor. Thank God Abigail came over and covered my legs with her husband's jacket. He proceeded to tell me to stay on the floor. While I am lying there, he begins to ask the crowd who knows this woman. The older couple said, "She's with us". He asked my name and they told him, "Venus... He said, her name is Venus!" Then he looked over at me and said these powerful, anointed words, "Venus, no knife will every touch your body, be healed, whether you think you deserve it or you don't believe you deserve it - you are healed." He told me to touch my breast and when I did, what I felt was astonishing - what was once a large mass was now very small. Praise God! Remarkable touch!

When I returned to my seat, I was so full of gratitude that I just kept crying and hugging Abigail. As ministry time and prayer continued, I decide to step out to the restroom to freshen up. As I was leaving, I saw Pastor Billy praying over Glenda, a beautiful lady with long black hair. As he was talking to her, she told him that she had stage 4 cancer. When I came back into the meeting room, Glenda was walking down the aisle to return to her seat, I paused for a moment to give her a hug, never saying a word to her.

At this point, Pastor Billy is going around the room, touching all the people on the forehead and I was not letting him forget about me! I start saying, Me, Me, Me next, Me Next... I'm not so sure what the Pastor thought of me, I didn't care, the presence of God was so strong that I wanted all I could get.

Some of you may be quite skeptical right now and wonder what does it mean to be "slain in the spirit". To be slain in the spirit you have to be willing to first yield to the Holy Spirit. As you stand waiting to be prayed for, turn your thoughts toward how good God is and how He gave His all for so that you might be made whole.

Being slain in the Spirit is simply when the presence and power of God comes onto you causing you to either fall forward or backward. His power can either come directly through the hands of someone operating under the Lord's anointing at any given moment, or directly at you by God Himself, such as when you see people falling to the ground while just sitting in their seats with no one laying a hand on them. Ezekiel 44:4 *"Then He brought me by way of the north gate to the front of the temple; so I looked, and behold, the glory of the Lord filled the house of the Lord; and* **I fell on my face.***"*

God is God. He can move and operate in whatever fashion He feels is necessary to bless us and heal us. I refuse to limit Him, nor will I doubt what He capable of doing. He is Creator, He is Savior, and He is Remarkable God.

It was so surreal when we left and returned to the hotel. I wrote down the words that were spoken over me that night to keep as a reminder of hope and encouragement. I slept like a baby. I normally do not sleep well in hotels because of the molds, dander in the rugs, bedding and air conditioning. But tonight the peace of God was hovering over me. Remarkable experience!

The next day when I was checking out of the hotel I ran into Glenda (the lady I saw in church last night) and her husband who was sporting several large crosses around his neck. She said "honey, this is the lady I was telling you about." What happened to me in church obviously affected the people that were there that evening. We formally introduced ourselves and she said, "Look what the chemo is doing to me – it's just brutal." Her husband interrupted us to tell me that he too has a healing ministry. They both have seen many miracles, but yet they were not allowing her be a miracle. Her husband began sharing a story about a woman who came to their church with a huge mass in her colon. It was so large that you could see it moving through the skin. After he prayed over her, she went into bathroom and the mass came out. When she returned her dress was hanging on her body. They have seen many miracles but not yet in Glenda's health. As I continued talking to her, I boldly said, "maybe you shouldn't have anymore chemo treatments, they are really making you sick, instead look to your great Physician, God." We exchanged contact information before I left and I followed up once with her to see how she was doing. She was very sick at the time. In my heart I don't know if she is still alive, but I certainly do hope and pray that she too receives a miracle as I did.

The next day I was excited to share the animated version of what had happened to me when Pastor Billy Burke prayed for me. To take my story to the next level, I decided to demonstrate the events of the evening for them. Teresa said this could be the end of the book! As I thought more about her statement, I paused to think...I believe this is not the ending – it's the beginning. Remarkable beginnings!

This entire experience has led me to do more research on Christian healers. Let me be clear here, I am not talking about metaphysical healers. I am talking about Christian men and women who are vessels that God uses to heal. All of this has opened my eyes to the world of the supernatural. I am constantly finding more and more fascinating information about God and healing. My confidence and faith continue to increase daily. If you like to read or listen to CD's, I recommend Gloria Copeland's healing teaching, (www.kcm.org), Healed of cancer by Dodie Osteen, all of the scriptures she stood on during her battle with cancer can be located on this website, (http://hopefaithprayer.com/scriptures/healing-scriptures-dodie-osteen/), and Andrew Womack (www.awmi.net) also has some wonderful teaching on healing.

My friendship with Teresa Tapp has continued to grow over the last couple of years. She invited me back to another T-Tapp event she was hosting. This time I perfected my speech and delivered some more great information to those who were in attendance. During this particular trip, I decided it was time to visit my parents. It's been nine years since I've seen my father. That's a long time to go without seeing someone. Something spectacular happened during my visit. I realized that I had completely forgiven him after all these years. It was one of the happiest times of my life. I was able to enjoy spending the day with both of my parents without any anxiety. There was laughter and a peace that hovered over me the entire time. A true remarkable healing of the heart had taken place.

I have to include this incredible doctor in this chapter! Dr. Rob Carlson, whom I met at a conference, changed my life! He has taught me about the importance in keeping your hormones balanced. He's actually a cardiologist, who is doing hormone work, specializing in treatment for women and really understands breast cancer. He has done wonders in balancing my hormones. One of the things I like most about him - is that he takes the time to thoroughly explain everything to you and answers all of your questions. I feel remarkable!

April 2011 *Well can it get any better than this? Remarkably Yes! I am feeling the urge to plan a trip to San Jose. I love California and I would love to see my dear friend, Jan Skuba, whom I have known since I was fifteen. Plus if you will remember from Good Friday, she is the one who put me in touch with the minister Eli. He and his wife prayed for me over the phone right after I was diagnosed. I really want to see Jan and meet Eli and his wife in person.*

My trip wasn't as long as I wished it could have been. During my stay, we made time to feed the homeless with Eli. After we finished working with those less fortunate, a group of us went back to Eli's home. Eli's wife had been healed from cancer after two years of trusting God and believing His word. By the time she went to the doctor, it was so severe that blood was oozing from her breast and it had metastasized to her brain. But she put her trust in God and by walking out her faith, God miraculously healed her.

While we were hanging out and discussing healing, Eli decides to pray for me. When he prayed, he spoke over my entire body. He prayed not only for me to be healed of cancer, but he prayed over all of my organs, ligaments and my back which went immediately into place. Needless to say, I was slain in the spirit. Good thing he asked me to stand by the sofa before he started praying. As I fell back, this awful sound came out of me, "Oof," and my friend Jan, said, "boo…ya!" Thinking back over this, it makes me laugh.

In closing out this chapter, I can tell you with confidence that I know I am healed. I am staying on the path and walking by faith each and everyday. I am excited about life and the future that God has in store for me. God told me that one day I would share my story to take the fear out of the hearts of others. I know that it's time to share the wealth of knowledge I have acquired on my journey. Remember the prayer partner from the earlier chapters? Well, another remarkable relationship came, by her praying for me.

As I began researching and talking to potential ghostwriters, I wasn't getting the responses I was looking for. One day God impressed upon my heart to ask Lisa to assist me. When I called her, she told me, that when she was praying, God told her to write, but she didn't know what that looked like, that was just two days prior to me calling her. I tell her all the time… she gets me! I find it amazing how God connected us from the beginning. Now, here we are at the beach compiling all the details of my story, what a remarkable journey! Remarkable, absolutely remarkable!

Remarkable Journey - Remarkable Relationships

Remarkable Experiences - Remarkable Knowledge

Venus DeMarco with Lisa Smith

Remarkable New Beginnings - Remarkable Future

Remarkable God - Remarkable

I feel Remarkable

"This is the day that the Lord has made, I will rejoice and be glad in it."

Psalm 118: 24

Laughter

We think of fun as a party—fun—being outdoors, being with family, beach outings, and vacation with family.

Webster defines laughter as an inner quality, mood, or disposition. I on the other hand define it as a good medicine to the heart and soul.

If I can give you some advice, don't ever become your disease. You can get so wrapped up in it that you stop living your life. I want to remind you that Cancer is just visiting. If you've put life on pause after being diagnosed, press the button and start living life large.

I am constantly reaching out to others that have been diagnosed, trying to share my insight and the things that I am learning along this journey. One day I invited a woman over to my apartment who was diagnosed with breast cancer. She told me that she literally thought about her treatments every single minute of the day. I remember telling her that,

"You are not your disease." And she said, "Yes, I am." She had become obsessed with the disease and was not living her life. Six months passed by and I ran into her one night when I was out. She asked what I had been doing and I told her that I had spent a fun evening at a wine bar with some of my friends. She replied, "What's fun? I don't remember…" She had forgotten how to enjoy her life. It could be as simple as reading a book, going to the movies, laughing with friend or having a glass of wine.

I will admit that in the beginning it was hard to have fun, trying to be perfect in all that I was doing. Great effort and constant thought was put into what I was eating, how much rest I was I getting, and remembering to take all my supplements consistently… I never knew how to be moderate with my always a bigger than life personality. I have traveled all over, had lots of lovers, I've been married, and I can party. There was no such thing as moderation to me. But I have learned in everything to apply moderation in order to bring good health and well being to my body and soul.

More powerful than expensive drugs! Did you know that people who laugh on a regular basis live longer, are healthier and make better decisions? Let's really look at laughter and humor a little closer, or if you haven't found a reason to laugh today, take a look in the mirror that should help. Humor people! *Proverbs 17:22 – "A cheerful mind works healing; a broken spirit dries up the bones."*

Every time we laugh it means we are getting healthier,

stronger, younger, smarter, and blessings are flowing through our system. It's the best stress reliever. Laughter lowers blood pressure, helps you get a good night's sleep, and it even increases your brain power. The best thing about laughter is it brings down walls and helps build relationships. In other words, humor opens up doors.

There is too much sadness in the world today, people are beaten down, let people hear your laughter, and there is healing in just hearing laughter. Let's be like children, when we were children we knew how to laugh. Let's release the child in us. God has given us everything we need to keep us healthy and whole, dust off your laughing machine. It will stimulate your immune system kick those NK cells (natural killer cells – they are the natural patrolman in our body. These natural killer cells eat bad things. They protect us from disease.

Negative emotions such as sadness, depression and anger slow the immune system way down. When we laugh we release the healing power that God placed inside of us. I've read of people who made sure that they only watched funny movies and stayed away from anything that brought out negative emotions like fear, healed very quickly, they kept their healing mechanism turned on. *Job 8:21 – "God wants to fill your mouth with laughter."*

People who laugh and have a good sense of humor and are easy to be around have more of the lovely NK cells. I miss sitting around telling jokes I still love to tell a good joke. It not only makes the person I'm telling it to laugh, but I crack myself up. So as it says in *Acts 20:24*

"We are to finish our course with joy."

If I Had to Do It Over Again

As they say hindsight is 20/20. I truly believe if I knew what I know now and had consistently practiced these habits starting many years ago, such as truly forgiving and making sure there was no anger in my heart, taking care of all those cellular memories that we don't even know we have, eating the proper alkaline plant based diet and exercising properly, I would not have had to live through the hell of a diagnosis of cancer. But with all that said if I hadn't taken this journey, my life might not have changed for the better and I would have missed the true kindness of the human race.

As I look back on my journey and all that I have experienced and learned, I could not be more grateful to have learned the truth. The truth is that God fearfully and wonderfully created the human body, so that it can heal itself from any disease. Knowledge is truth! Knowing what I know now, this is the plan I would make for myself if I was diagnosed today.

The best part of this is I could bypass all the time I wasted on fear. My body would have been spared the mental and physical effect that the fear of the diagnosis does to the body. First and most importantly, I would get into agreement with God's promises for me and receive His healing for me. As Andrew Womack says, *"It's a combination of grace and faith that releases the power of God. Grace is God's part and faith is defined as being a positive response to what God has already provided by grace. Faith is your positive response to God's grace."*

Secondly, I would have rescheduled my clients for the next three weeks, found a place for my dog to stay, and I would have checked myself into one of the following health establishments that are known for getting you into the state of optimal health; such as the Hippocrates Health Institute in Florida, The Optimal Health Institute (OHI) located in Texas and California, or The Gerson Institute in Mexico. You will find that there are many alternative places to choose from.

The purpose for getting away is to eliminate stress, calm yourself physically and emotionally as well as get your body into an alkaline state; while being away from your family, friends and your job and most importantly their fear. Another wonderful benefit of these places is that they prepare your food, juices and treat your needs accordingly.

By taking this first step I believe I would have saved a lot of money in the long run. After my stay I would have already been through some of the detox process, gotten in an alkaline state and received key information from these experts which would have allowed me to relax a lot sooner. When I returned home I would have found a local naturopathic doctor to work with in case I need additional advice and/or treatments.

Knowing what I know, I believe the journey would have been much shorter in receiving my healing and a clean bill of health. But I would have missed some of the interesting situations I experienced along my journey.

I would of still purchased a Vita Mix and a juicer and set my kitchen up for my new healthier way of eating. I'm doing this without stress and fear because I know my body can heal itself from any past damage and will remain healthy and cancer free. Nahum 1:9 – *"Affliction will not rise up a second time."* If you will take the time and do your homework, you will find that there is a lot of amazing information out there about the natural cures for cancer.

If your healing isn't manifested immediately, keep walking in blind faith, then choose one protocol and stick to it and allow your body to heal. It's up to each of us to take responsibility for our bodies. I Corinthians 6:19 (MSG) - *"Or didn't you realize that your body is a sacred place, the place of the Holy Spirit? Don't you see that you can't live however you please; squandering what God paid such a high price for? The physical part of you is not some piece of property belonging to the spiritual part of you. God owns the whole works. So let people see God in and through your body."*

When you get your clean bill of health don't get lazy, stay with this new lifestyle and live a long healthy life in the name of Jesus. My wish for you is to realize that God has designed a miracle for everyone. Just ask for it, it has your name on it. Your miracle is right around the corner. Just claim it!

"I wait for the Lord. I shall change and renew my strength and power. I shall lift my wings and mount up as eagles. I shall run and not be weary; I shall walk and not faint or become tired."
Isaiah 40:31